D1547152

The How-to Guide to Home Health Therapy Documentation

CINDY KRAFFT, PT, MS

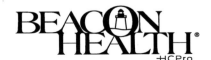

BEAC☉N
HEALTH®
+HCPro

The How-to Guide to Home Health Therapy Documentation is published by Beacon Health, a division of HCPro, Inc.

Copyright © 2011 Beacon Health, a division of HCPro, Inc.

Cover Image © Nicemonkey. Used under license from Shutterstock.com.

Download the additional materials of this book at *www.hcpro.com/downloads/9405*.

ISBN: 978-1-60146-830-7

HCPro, Inc., provides information resources for the healthcare industry.

HCPro, Inc., is not affiliated in any way with The Joint Commission, which owns the JCAHO and Joint Commission trademarks.

Cindy Krafft, PT, MS, Author
Adrienne Trivers, Managing Editor
Jamie Carmichael, Associate Group Publisher
Emily Sheahan, Group Publisher
Mike Mirabello, Senior Graphic Artist
Matt Sharpe, Production Supervisor
Shane Katz, Art Director
Jean St. Pierre, Senior Director of Operations

Advice given is general. Readers should consult professional counsel for specific legal, ethical, or clinical questions. Arrangements can be made for quantity discounts. For more information, contact:

Beacon Health, a division of HCPro, Inc.
75 Sylvan Street, Suite A-101
Danvers, MA 01923
Telephone: 800/650-6787 or 781/639-1872
Fax: 800/639-8511
E-mail: *customerservice@hcpro.com*

Visit Beacon Health online at: *www.beaconhealth.org*

05/2011
21889

Contents

CONTENTS

The How-to Guide to Home Health Therapy Documentation

CONTENTS

CONTENTS

About the Author

Cindy Krafft, PT, MS

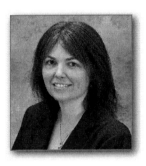

Cindy Krafft, PT, MS, is the director of rehabilitation consulting services for Fazzi Associates, Inc. She has 16 years of home health experience ranging from PRN clinician to the director of rehabilitation for a six-agency home-care system. She serves as the president of the Home Health Section of the American Physical Therapy Association (APTA) and the chair of the NAHC Therapy Advisory Committee. Krafft is the codirector of the Delta Excellence in Therapy Project completed in September 2010. She has been published in *Caring* magazine, *Remington Report, Success in Home Care, Home Healthcare Nurse,* and the newsletter of the Home Health Section of APTA.

As well as being an expert on therapy practice in homecare, Krafft assists agencies with OASIS competency. She served as the clinical codirector of Delta National OASIS-C Best Practices Project. She has been a well-received speaker at both the state and national levels on the topics of OASIS and therapy documentation, program development, therapy utilization, and recruitment. She currently works with agencies on developing their rehabilitation programs, training staff and management on appropriate therapy documentation, and providing therapy documentation audits so agencies can effectively navigate regulations and protect payment.

Cindy lives with her husband Walter and their four children Adam, Joshua, Nathan, and Sarah. She began her career in home health to spend more time with them and credits their continued support as the driving force behind her determination to be a consistent advocate for patients and caregivers.

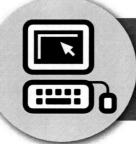

DOWNLOAD YOUR MATERIALS NOW

For additional materials on home health documentation go to the website listed below.

www.hcpro.com/downloads/9405

Thank you for purchasing this product!

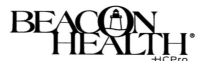

Welcome to the World of Home Health

For some it is a deliberate plan. Others enter this arena initially as a side job or a way to make a little extra money. Some may wonder how they ended up here at all. Regardless of the route, more and more therapists are finding themselves as part of the home health community both in a clinical capacity as well as in leadership roles. With respect to preparation, many therapists have had little to no exposure to home health as part of their educational curriculum. After accepting a position with an agency or contract company, far too many have limited or scattered orientation to this setting and can experience the frustration of not understanding the unique expectations that surround this area of practice. The phrase "I just wanted to do therapy" has been uttered in agencies large and small across the country and, in some cases, has been the reason good clinicians throw in the towel and change clinical settings. The vision of being surrounded by roaches in less than desirable neighborhoods and spending time drowning in paperwork is how many therapists view home health from the outside looking in. The brave souls that stay in this setting know the fundamental truth that keeps them going out every day: the ability to directly impact the quality of life for patients in a very real way. The documentation challenges in this setting are significant, yet there are limited sources of information to guide the home health therapist to meet the demands of the payer sources and the agencies—until now.

Home Health Prospective Payment System

Prior to 2000, home health agencies were paid by Medicare on a per visit basis. There was a set dollar amount for each discipline and, as long as "skilled" issues were present, care could go on unabated. It was not unusual to have patients on service continuously for literally years at a time. Discharge planning was not clear and many patients expected to be the ones to decide when they were finished with the services. This care delivery model was generating many visits and in most cases satisfied patients, but there was no consistent measurable way to determine the impact of the care being provided. If left on its own, each agency could make up its own assessment tools following the regulations as a guide, but the end result was as many different tools as there were agencies. In order to gather standardized and consistent data, the Outcome and Assessment Information Set (OASIS) instrument was created with nationwide implementation in agencies on January 1, 2000. The focus of the tool is outcome measurement, as the name implies, but it was selected for a secondary purpose. Because every agency in the country was going to use it, the decision was made to use some of the questions to determine payment for the care provided. In addition to the more clinically driven items, a new one was added specifically for payment—MO825—and the relationship between the number of therapy visits and reimbursement was born.

There are more payer sources for home health besides Medicare, with private insurance, Medicaid, and HMOs involved to varying degrees depending on the region of the country. Medicare, both traditional and managed, remains the largest driver of home health practice, and additional third party payers are moving to the Medicare episodic model of payment. That being said, references to Medicare may appear a narrow focus at first glance, but the key concepts apply to the provision of home health regardless of the source of payment.

Along with OASIS came the model of the 60-day episode for home health. As long as the patient qualifies for services, he or she is allowed to continue, but formal reassessments were now expected if care was going to extend beyond 60 days. Essentially the industry was placed on a budget, with OASIS used to calculate the dollar amount associated with the individual patient and the Home Health Prospective Payment System (PPS) era began. One of the goals was to eliminate what previously appeared to be an incentive to keep visiting patients when being paid by the visit. Within the model, there was a piece of the puzzle that looked and felt like a per visit model in relation to the provision of therapy.

Initially, the model added approximately $2,200 to the payment for the episode if the patient was in need of 10 or more therapy visits. This was calculated as any combination of therapy visits or any therapy alone that would reach that number. The decision to select 10 as the threshold was based on industry data that, at the time, indicated the peak number of therapy visits was five to seven, so 10 was not considered a routine occurrence. The intent was to provide appropriate resources to support patients whose level of care exceeded what was routinely being provided. If the needs of the patient were the sole driver of therapy practice pattern at the time, one would expect it to be virtually unchanged by the implementation of a PPS. That was not the case.

Changes in Therapy Practice Patterns

Medicare continued to analyze visit data for all home health services and, after a few years in the prospective payment model, noticed that therapy visit patterns appeared to be changing. The shift was upward with more and more patients now receiving 10 or more therapy visits and agencies reaching the payment threshold that came along with it. Data reflects that at one point more than 50% of the time agencies responded on OASIS that the threshold would be met and the total number of visits ended between 10 and 13—a very different pattern than prior to the year 2000.

The Medicare response to this came in 2008 when the therapy threshold was replaced with a tiered model. The intent was to better align payment with a wider range of visit numbers as opposed to a single threshold. The relationship between therapy visits and payment remained and has followed a tiered model since implementation on January 1, 2008. Once again, expectations were that therapy practice would remain fairly stable in light of this payment model change, but the visit data does not appear to validate that idea.

When putting together the PPS update for 2011, Medicare references a 26% increase in patients receiving 14 or more therapy visits. This shift upward began shortly after the model change that created significant increases in reimbursement when more than 14 total therapy visits are provided to the patient. Some have wondered why there is that kind of payment increase at specifically the 14th visit as therapists will clearly state there is no clinical relevance to that particular number. The selection was based on the visit data of the industry. Updated PPS data showed the majority of home health patients received 13 visits or fewer, with 14 to 19 being infrequent and 20 or more rarely done. A second practice pattern change appearing to be correlated to an adjustment in the payment structure has raised the concerns of many, both within the industry as well as outside entities.

Validating the medical necessity of therapy services is driven by documentation. This is true for all healthcare settings, with some getting more attention than others. Therapists that have come from the acute care setting, for example, may reminisce about how much less documentation they had to do when compared to home health. This has led to the perception that home health has very different expectations, but in reality this is not the case. The current level of scrutiny on home health therapy documentation is a direct result of the relationship between the number of therapy visits and reimbursement, which has a higher direct level of impact when compared to other settings. When combined with not one but two apparent practice pattern shifts, one can clearly see why Medicare and others are so interested in the documentation specifics. Practicing in the home setting carries with it the expectation to show why the patient needed the services and what the clinicians did for and to the patient that could not be done by another discipline or a lay person.

"Fixing" Therapy Documentation

One could simply try to create a list of words or phrases that the therapists could pick from to "improve" documentation without much effort. Some have tried this route but success is limited. Content tends to become repetitive quickly and lacks patient specificity as well as a clear picture of the involvement of the therapists. Before getting into the details of documentation content, it is important for the therapist to get a larger perspective on this unique practice setting as this helps to explain the "why" behind the expectations and empowers therapists with a working knowledge of how to clearly document the necessary information.

Time to Make a Choice

One can argue that therapists are making practice decisions that they know were never influenced by the reimbursement model. This is true in the majority of agencies, and the needs of the patient should always be the driving force of decision-making. However, some have been influenced either blatantly or more subtly, and the end result is data that calls what is being done by all three therapies into question.

The time has passed to debate what is "fair" or "unfair" in all of this. Therapists know the patients need their services but feel overwhelmed and frustrated with getting it down on paper or into a computer. In desperation they say, "just tell me what you want me to put down." The time has come to change how therapy documentation and care delivery is viewed in the home health setting. Change is not easy but at times it is necessary.

Documentation has to get back under the control of the therapists with a clear orientation to how to create meaningful content in a time-efficient manner with the focus remaining on the patient. At the end of the day, the patient is the primary reason any therapist stays in the home health setting, and effective documentation has to be embraced as a critical element of excellent patient care.

Documentation: The "D" Word

People generally choose to enter a healthcare profession based on a desire to help others. Regardless of practice setting, documentation is often seen as a necessary evil that comes along with the profession and is not often viewed in a positive light. Any discussion of documentation tends to provoke feelings of frustration and the assumption that high-quality content must require a large volume of both detail and time. In order to better understand these concerns, it is important to look at how therapists learn to document the care they provide.

Back to the Beginning

When starting out in a physical therapy, occupational therapy, or speech-language pathology educational program, students typically have a limited working knowledge of clinical skills and documentation. As patient care skills are acquired, each instructor has expectations as to the content of documentation that should be created based on simulated patient situations. Students learn quickly that each instructor has a slightly, or not so slightly, different style and, in order to be successful in a specific class, the documentation needs to comply with those expectations. In order to meet the goal of becoming a therapist, students can become conditioned from early in their educational experience that documentation is generated based on the needs of someone else and is not really of value to them personally. This is reinforced during early clinical experiences when the student is excited to be practicing his or her newly acquired skills on real people.

When documenting this care, it must meet the expectations of the individual clinical instructor in order to meet the ultimate goals of graduation and licensure. When finally out on their own, therapists are told that the payer source has expectations for content in order to pay for services rendered. In order to truly impact the quality of clinical documentation, therapists need to start with a clean slate and reorient themselves to the importance of this area of practice.

Documentation in Home Health

Home health has the reputation of having a lot of paperwork, and this has been an obstacle, at times, to successful recruitment of staff. Progress in technology has brought laptop computers to the bedside, which has reduced the physical nature of carrying around stacks of paper, but the apparent volume of work seems to increase with each passing year. Layer upon layer piles up until it seems that there is no possible way to be compliant with all of the rules and regulations combined with agency practice and the specific demands of the software system. In comparison, documentation expectations in the hospital or outpatient setting seem not only significantly lower but also much less time-consuming for the clinicians to complete effectively and efficiently.

Practicing in a "clinic without walls" has provided flexibility in scheduling the activities of the day, and documentation is very often left until the end and sometimes well into the evening after family commitments are addressed. Concerns regarding the amount of time spent and the intrusion on personal time are fairly routine occurrence for home health clinicians—nurses and therapists alike. It is a viable question to wonder why there are so many expectations specific to home health.

As mentioned in the previous chapter, home health has a history with respect to therapy practice patterns that has raised concerns about what truly motivates the number of visits provided. The data suggests that the reimbursement structure appears to be a contributing factor in the eyes of Medicare. Interactions with therapy in the form of minutes spent, visits made, or units provided have impact on payment received in various healthcare settings.

When comparing the impact of the provision of therapy on reimbursement in the hospital setting, it is much less direct and a significantly lower percentage of the total payment for care than it is in home health. Concerns regarding the medical necessity of care tend to escalate the more the financial relevance to ensure care delivery is based on patient need and not a perceived incentive to provide any specific discipline or disciplines. This has been translated into the appearance of higher demands on the content of therapy notes in home health as opposed to the hospital where a visit note may be a few sentences instead of several pages. Even within the home health arena, there is more discussion about and external scrutiny of the content of physical therapy, occupational therapy, and speech-language pathology notes than on those generated by nurses, medical social workers, and home health aides. The need to be clear as to the condition of the patient and the skilled interventions being provided is of equal importance regardless of setting or discipline because it defines and supports each profession as vitally important to the driving force of care—the patient.

In a facility setting, many tasks can be divided among disciplines or departments. Getting consents, securing orders, completing the comprehensive assessment, reviewing medications, and dealing with psychosocial issues are examples of tasks that tend to fall to different disciplines to take the lead within the hospital or skilled nursing facility yet can fall to one person or discipline within home health.

Documenting these activities is an integral part of home health care yet it is very often the detail that is left out of the notes and has created records that appear to have limited skilled content. Annual payment reductions from Medicare have become a way of life for home health agencies, and it has been implied that care is being overprovided, with visits being made to people who do not really need care. The industry responds with frustration and outrage and insists that providing care to this particular population requires more resources, not less, as patients present with more issues and a higher acuity level than in years past. Lack of detail in the documentation equates to not taking credit for the complexity of both the patient and the care provided.

Documentation tools

The documentation tools available to home health therapists are often considered to be a contributing factor to issues with content. Therapists throughout the country express varying degrees of concerns and frustration with the forms they are asked to use. This is not limited to paper or to electronic options because both present opportunities and challenges when trying to document skilled care. Some key areas are outlined in Figure 2.1.

FIGURE 2.1	Documentation tools

Paper Tools

Pros	Cons
Changes and updates can be made internally at the agency level	Legibility can be an issue
Documentation flow can move around the sheets of paper with ease	Accessibility by other clinicians is difficult
Allow for narrative information to be added as needed	Papers can be lost, misplaced, or incorrectly filed
Can physically hold the forms which is a preference of some therapists	Physical challenge of carrying multiple forms and making copies

Electronic Tools

Pros	Cons
Legibility is good regardless of the clinician doing the documentation	Changes and updates often require vendor involvement and can be delayed
Other disciplines and clerical staff can access notes	Layout forces documentation to be completed in a more standard order
Additional copies can be printed if paper version has been misplaced	Reliance on drop-down options alone with limited narrative capacity
Convenience of having access to all necessary forms in one place	Challenge of learning to use the technology effectively

With respect to tools, there are issues no matter what the format. The responsibility of providing documentation content that clearly supports medical necessity falls squarely on the shoulders of the therapists, and gaps cannot be blamed on any specific tool issues. The therapist must be diligent in creating appropriate detail that is a balance of "check boxes" and narrative content to show the individuality of each patient. As an example, the documentation tool may lack a specific designated area for prior level of function. All three therapy disciplines have been taught that this is a key piece of information as part of an assessment yet an individual therapist chooses to not document any detail on that subject because there "wasn't a place for it."

During an audit, the lack of prior level of function content raises concern because there is now no clear way to determine the baseline performance of the patient upon which goals were supposed to be built. Other chapters in this book examine documentation content more closely, but therapists must understand that the tools they are given to use will not stand up as an excuse as to why good content was not seen in the notes.

Completing documentation

A frequent strategy for managing the paperwork in home health is to defer documentation until the end of the day or the following day. This can allow for therapists to be home at a reasonable time and be available for personal events. At face value, this seems like an effective plan, but one has to question the impact on accuracy of the information being recorded. Meaningful key details can be lost in the time between the care delivery and the note generation, especially when multiple visits have been completed during that time. As an example, think about the first person you encountered yesterday. Can a detailed description of what he or she was wearing, hair and eye color, and the first words spoken be accurately generated? One can argue that, without a plan to remember all of that information, some aspects of the description may be omitted now. If there was a plan, clarity would improve by jotting down a few cues to refer to later.

In the context of a busy day doing patient visits, critical elements like the verbal cues provided during training or the recommendation made to the patient's daughter can be overlooked when starting from scratch several hours later. When calculating the average length of a visit, historically about 45 minutes for all three therapies, Medicare assumes and expects that documentation is part of that time. No one is suggesting that the patient should be set up in front of the television while the therapist documents for a half an hour but, when none of it is done during the time of the visit, the end result is a shorter visit and the possibility of less accurate content. Specific to the Outcome and Assessment Information Set, completion of the tool in the presence of the patient is expected in order to ensure accurate data collection. Therapists need to recognize the importance of this as part of care delivery and understand that documentation as part of the visit is critical to creating the level of detail necessary to support medical necessity.

Making Peace

No one would suggest that documentation is delightful and that therapists will learn to love it. However, some level of peace and acceptance must be reached in order to move past the current environment of confusing and conflicting information as well as the frustration that is leading to insufficient content. High-quality assessments, visit notes, and clinical summaries are not about the amount of information that is written but are driven by the focus of the content to clearly support medical necessity. Mythical lists of the correct statements to use to ensure payment are not the answer. The level of detail needed to support the ongoing inclusion of physical therapy, occupational therapy, and speech-language pathology as integral parts of home health care requires therapists to regain ownership of this important issue and revisit what they know to be skilled care.

Medical Necessity

Understanding Medical Necessity

Much like the age old debate about which came first, the chicken or the egg, home health therapists need to determine the relationship between patient care and documentation. As long as any therapist can remember, the statement, "If you didn't document it, you didn't do it" has been used to the point at which it has lost actual meaning. Does documentation drive the skilled care being delivered or is it the other way around? It can easily feel like documentation comes first with all of the attention being paid to therapy utilization with medical necessity being defined by the level of content seen in every individual patient encounter.

The search for the "right" way to record skilled care appears elusive and has led to myths and apparent quick fixes to address concerns. One of the largest myths of all with respect to therapy documentation is that progress equals skilled care. Although it is true that the patient should show positive impact from the interventions provided, these changes alone do not, in and of themselves, support the need for therapy to be involved in the plan of care. This is not an issue of terminology but of focus.

The term "medical necessity" is used often in healthcare but can lack clarity to the individual clinician. It is helpful to consider the dictionary definition of the word necessity—which contains a very helpful piece of the puzzle—indispensability. The fact that a person has a medical condition such as congestive heart failure does not automatically mean that nursing or therapy services are warranted. There are plenty of people of Medicare age with the diagnosis of heart failure, diabetes, or peripheral vascular disease that are not in need of skilled care. That being said, accurate diagnosis coding is a critical element of the home health admission assessment because it communicates the complexity of the patients being served to Medicare and other payers. The support for necessity is driven by what the individual discipline can provide to a patient that could not be done as well or at all by another discipline, a family member, or caregiver. The medical condition can set the stage, but the key element is defining what the specific discipline—physical therapy, occupational therapy, or speech-language pathology—is going to provide to the patient that will have a meaningful impact. Progress in the traditional sense may occur because of these interventions but will not stand alone to show skill.

A great example of the "need" for therapy is the orthopedic patient. When a person has a knee replaced or has fallen and broken a hip, the inclusion of therapy services in the plan of care is expected. There is little to no debate with the physician as to whether or not therapy will be ordered and, overwhelmingly, the service included most often is physical therapy. Why would a knee replacement mean physical therapy is warranted? Does the implant drive it? Do the surgical procedure and the subsequent incision line require the attention of a therapist? The expectation is the therapist will address range of motion, strength, balance, and gait deficits that have been impacted by the knee replacement using specific techniques that are uniquely physical therapy. If a nurse or the patient's daughter could provide the exact same level of care, there would be no logical reason for therapy to be involved. It is not the medical condition alone that supports the necessity of care but the impact one or more of these conditions may have on a patient's ability to function that requires intervention from a skilled therapist to improve.

There has been a fundamental communication gap between nurses and therapists when developing a plan of care. This is why the classic answer to the question, "How many therapy visits would a patient with heart failure need?" is almost always answered with a variation of "it depends." The diagnosis label triggers a set of possible interventions that nursing will bring to the table. That same label is not enough information by itself to establish the therapy component. The therapist will want to know what specifically has been impacted with respect to function, and to what extent, before determining a course of action. Those differences must be kept in mind as it is the unique interventions that support medical necessity. Without that information, the notes appear to be repeated assessments and do not show what the therapist was doing with and for the patient that precipitated changes to occur.

Looking at it a different way

Here is another way to think about it. Imagine that when you woke up this morning and headed to the bathroom to get ready for the day, water was all over the floor. This is not a little puddle but enough that you knew something was wrong. You have to get to work and already have a busy day planned so time is short to deal with this situation. A call is made to your good friend who is married to a plumber and you ask the plumber to come over during the day to fix the problem. (For the sake of argument, in this example, you are not secretly a plumber or particularly handy.) At the end of yet another hectic day of seeing patients, you arrive home and go straight to the bathroom. Happily, there is no longer any water on the floor, indicating progress has occurred. The situation has improved compared to what it was that very morning. On the counter there is a slip of paper representing the bill for the services provided. It reads: "It was broken. I am a plumber, and I fixed it. Total cost is $1,500."

There is little that would make anyone excited about paying $1,500 for anything, but there is clearly not enough information in that note to justify the amount. Key items missing are what the problem actually was, how long the plumber was working on it, what parts were involved, and what had to be done to install them. Bottom line, you would want to see enough detail to indicate that you could not have taken care of the problem yourself for a lesser cost. At an even more basic level, how do you know the plumber did not just mop up the water and leave? It is very frustrating to realize that you paid someone to do something that did not actually require a specific set of skills. Connecting this to documentation in healthcare, why do nurses and therapists continue to submit notes that essentially read: "The patient was sick. I visited him. He is better now. Here is the bill."? The missing pieces are similar in that the therapist must show more than the end result of the care and be clear about what skilled interventions were utilized to achieve those goals. If you would not accept less from a plumber in your home, why do we expect less from ourselves when documenting the care we provide?

An extension of the progress myth is the idea that a plateau means the patient has to be discharged. Some agencies have created practice patterns around this idea and state that if progress is not seen in three visits, then the patient must be discharged as this is no longer skilled care. The lack of progress is not the dominant factor that defines the time to discontinue a skilled service. The decision to discharge is driven by the determination that there is nothing left for the specific discipline to contribute in terms of interventions that will benefit the patient. The idea that a patient can make clearly measurable improvements on every single visit is not realistic when considering the patient population we serve. This may be why therapy notes often appear to have arbitrary gains in ambulation of five to 10 feet or in repetitions of exercises on every visit as if that alone will demonstrate skilled care. When medical necessity is viewed from the standpoint of indispensability, it highlights the importance of detailed interventions in conjunction with progress that supports the inclusion of therapy services in the plan of care. When analyzing the typical course of care, plateaus happen periodically over the entire episode. The reason skilled care continues is the expectation that improvements will happen over time because there is more to be taught or techniques to be applied to this specific patient situation by each discipline involved. This concept is reinforced in the Home Health Prospective Payment System (PPS) updates for 2011 in relation to therapy reassessments. One purpose of the reassessment is to support why each therapy should continue providing care. There is no mention of this being solely supported by measurable progress or that lack of progress requires discharge. The documentation of the reassessment must contain a clinically supported statement of expectation that the patient can continue to progress or resume progress after plateau or regression. This confirms that Medicare is not the one dictating the discussion about progress equaling skilled care but a lack of clarity surrounding what the provision of skilled care actually is.

Transient and Easily Reversible

Medicare coverage criteria for home health contains the following statement: "Therapy would not be covered to effect improvement or restoration of function when a patient suffered a transient and easily reversible loss or reduction of function." It is interesting to note how many agencies have interpreted this as an issue of patient diagnosis and attempt to develop criteria to prevent "inappropriate" referrals from being made to physical therapy, occupational therapy, and speech-language pathology. Determination of the need for skilled therapy still rests with the therapist and is not based on any particular diagnosis. Even the most seasoned therapist may not see a patient's condition as transient on the first encounter. Nearly every home health therapist has been in some variation of the following situations.

- It is a lovely Friday morning. Upon arriving at the home, the therapist is met by a distraught patient's granddaughter who is overwhelmed with the amount of assistance her grandfather needs. She reports he was taking care of himself and getting around "pretty well" before he went to the hospital, but since returning home he has required a lot more help. The assessment reveals that the patient requires moderate assistance for ambulation, dressing, and toileting and maximum assistance for bathing, thereby indicating that both physical and occupational therapy will be part of the plan of care. Given the degree of decline since hospitalization, the physical therapist designs a plan that will require a significant amount of visits over the next few weeks—the plan is based on her clinical findings as well the goals of the patient and granddaughter to return to prior level of function. A basic home program is initiated as part of the evaluation visit. When the physical therapist returns for the next scheduled visit on Monday, the patient appears considerably better—more than the therapist would have expected at this point. The patient and granddaughter report that he ate well, slept much better in his own bed than at the hospital, and is really enjoying seeing his dog again whom he missed terribly when he was away. The patient reports he got up to walk several times a day to let the dog outside without any issues. Reassessment of the patient confirms he is able to function at a higher level than the previous week and, although he still requires some interventions from physical therapy, the plan will be adjusted to decrease the visits as the original number is no longer required. Does this physical therapist have magic powers or the ability to create home programs with special qualities to create this level of improvement OR could being back in the home environment have played a role in the patient's progress?

- On the other side of town on the same day, an occupational therapist is completing an evaluation of a patient who has been diagnosed with heart failure within the past month. The patient reports she is completing her self-care activities without "much help" from her husband as she prides herself in being very independent. The assessment reveals that the patient does not have any equipment in the bathroom to make bathing and toilet transfers less stressful. When completing these tasks without the equipment, the patient becomes mildly short of breath and tries to hurry. The occupational therapist recommends a transfer bench and a raised toilet seat to the patient who insists she is currently "fine," stating "I do not want that stuff in my house. My husband can help me." They discuss basic energy conservation strategies, and the patient seems agreeable but in a hurry to get through the material. She tells the occupational therapist that there are "too many people" coming in and out of her home since she returned there two days ago. She does not think she wants or needs therapy—especially since she already agreed to physical therapy and that "should be enough for me." The patient appears to be doing okay at this point, but the occupational therapist still has concerns. Based on these concerns, and taking into consideration the comments made by the patient, the occupational therapist presents a plan of care that would schedule the next visit in about two weeks to determine if things are continuing to go well or if additional interventions are necessary. When making that second visit, the therapist is pleasantly surprised to see a seat in the shower. The patient reports her daughter picked it up yesterday for her as she was just getting "too tired" when trying to bathe. The occupational therapist practices with the patient and instructs her how to safely use the seat and confirms that no additional intervention is needed with bathing or for the toilet transfer as the patient is doing well. The discharge is completed as there is no longer a need for a skilled occupational therapist to be involved in the plan of care. With the patient doing pretty well at the evaluation and concerned about the number of people in the home, the therapist could have misinterpreted "transient" and felt that no additional visits should be made—but that is incorrect based on the clinical findings and safety concerns that were noted. An additional visit or two to confirm the initial appearance of a patient with few needs as on the best path to safe function is considered skilled care and is a covered service.

These examples confirm that the determination of the need for therapy is not an issue of patient diagnosis or better screening prior to referral but the active participation of a skilled therapist making decisions about interventions needed by each individual patient. As the patient situation can change over the course of care, it is the therapist who must make adjustments based on clinical findings and not a formula or reference sheet, and the documentation generated by these activities is what supports the medical necessity of the care.

Maintenance Therapy

Any discussion of medically necessary therapy must include the topic of "maintenance therapy." Updates to Home Health PPS have drawn attention to this issue, and there has been some confusion and misunderstanding about how this concept fits into this practice setting. The end result has been the belief that maintenance therapy is a "new" area of growth for home health agencies and the feeling that Medicare has expanded coverage—neither of these is accurate. The definition of skilled therapy applies here as well because it must be clear that the skills of a therapist are indispensable to the patient.

MEDICAL NECESSITY

Delivery of therapy in the home setting falls into two general categories and both are defined by their focus. "Restorative" therapy is based on the intention to see improvements in the functional status of the patient as a result of skilled interventions. Keep in mind how improvement is measured as this is not a progress equal to skilled care discussion. The changes in the patient would impact the quality or quantity or both areas of functional performance in ways that are meaningful to the patient and reflect his or her participation in the plan of care. "Maintenance" therapy is used in situations where the assessment of the patient situation would indicate that substantial improvements are not expected and the focus is on prevention of decline. The plan of care is created with the intention of turning follow-through over to a nonskilled person like a family member or paid caregiver.

There are two different situations that meet the criteria of covered maintenance therapy in home health.

- **Situation 1:** It is determined that the patient is not going to show significant improvement and would not meet the intent of restorative therapy. The patient requires the skills of a therapist to make this determination, establish the necessary program, train the appropriate caregiver(s), and make any modifications to the program as indicated. Given the level of skill needed for all of these tasks, only a physical therapist, an occupational therapist, or a speech-language pathologist can perform these visits—therapist assistants cannot participate in the plan of care. In the language of the Medicare manual, covered maintenance therapy would "require the specialized skills, knowledge, and judgment of the qualified therapist to design or establish a safe and effective maintenance program."

  - **Example A:** A 68-year-old woman with long-standing heart failure is referred to occupational therapy to address limited ability to perform bathing and dressing safely. The occupational therapist completes the initial assessment and determines that the patient is current performing these tasks at the same level she has for the last three years but is concerned that she may decline if she does not stay active in self-care. Her daughter is very helpful—sometimes too helpful—and needs to know how to best assist her mom without facilitating additional dependence. The occupational therapist puts together a plan to educate the daughter and initiates a set of activities to keep the patient involved in her care. After a few visits, the occupational therapist is confident the patient and daughter have mastered the program and discharges them with the instruction to keep working on the tasks and strategies that were taught.

— **Example B:** An 85-year-old man with peripheral vascular disease is referred to physical therapy with concerns regarding his ability to safely get up from his chair and ambulate. The physical therapist assesses the patient and determines that his potential for significant improvement is low and sees the need to initiate a plan of care focused on teaching him and his wife strategies to decrease the difficulty of the transfer by increasing the height of the seating surface as well as a daily walking program to prevent further decline. The physical therapist completes several visits focused on education on these issues and to assess the patient's ability to tolerate a walking program. Once these tasks are mastered, the physical therapist discharges and instructs the patient and his wife to walk in the apartment complex at least once per day.

+ **Situation 2:** It is determined that the patient is not going to show significant improvement and would not meet the intent of restorative therapy. The patient requires the skills of a therapist to make this determination, establish the necessary program, train the appropriate caregiver(s), and make any modifications to the program as indicated. The complexity of the patient and/or the program being implemented indicates that it would not be safe to turn the care over to a nontherapist. Based on that determination, delivery of the maintenance program would be done by the therapist because there would be the need for ongoing assessments and modifications to the program based on the condition of the patient. This level of complexity indicates that all visits must be performed by the physical therapist, the occupational therapist, or the speech-language pathologist—therapy assistants cannot participate in the plan of care. In addition to the language of the Medicare manual noted for Situation 1, the following is taken into consideration here: "the unique clinical conditions of a patient may require the specialized skills of a qualified therapist to perform a safe and effective maintenance program."

— **Example C:** A 72-year-old woman with a history of a stroke about three years ago is referred to speech therapy because of concerns over her ability to safely handle thin liquids. The speech-language pathologist determines during the assessment that the patient has been using thickener as ordered but increased fatigue from her recent open heart surgery has impacted her swallowing inconsistently. The speech-language pathologist is concerned that the patient's new caregiver is having trouble remembering how to correctly cue and monitor the patient and establishes a plan of care to see the patient to monitor her thickener use and confirm the ability of the caregiver to assist. In a few weeks, the speech-language pathologist is confident the patient is managing well and discharges her on her original diet, now confident that the caregiver is able to follow through correctly.

— **Example D:** A 50-year-old woman with multiple sclerosis is referred to physical therapy to assess functional status after a recent hospitalization. Changes in the medication while in the hospital have impacted her ability to safely ambulate the limited distance she is capable of from her bedroom to the patio. She currently completes that distance, but the physical therapist determines that her ability to do this depends on the timing of her medication, which the nurse says are still being adjusted. There is a competent caregiver, but the physical therapist knows he will have to monitor this patient closely and adjust his recommended activities based on her overall status for the time being. Once the medication issues stabilize, so does the patient's functional abilities, and the physical therapist is now comfortable turning over follow-through to the caregiver and discharges the patient.

It is clear that the medical necessity component of maintenance therapy is the need for a skilled therapist to assess the patient, establish the plan of care, train the caregiver, and determine when the therapist is no longer indispensable. The care itself can be delivered and covered when the complexity of the patient or program means a therapist must be involved. Once again, skilled need is based on the nature of the interventions and the level of assessment and reassessment required by the patient. Maintenance therapy is not covered when the therapist is no longer contributing anything meaningful to the plan of care because visits have become repetitive in nature and no variation is seen in the interventions being utilized.

Therapists may struggle internally with the patient they know is not going to follow through on recommendations or will not do the exercises unless someone comes and tells them to. They know that it is very likely the patient will decline and a new referral may be made. Logic would indicate that simply keeping this patient on service would be better than discharging, but the Medicare benefit does not cover that as medically necessary therapy as there is no need for the specific skills of a therapist for that level of care.

Defining Skilled Care

Therapists have spent far too long looking to external sources to define what skilled physical therapy, occupational therapy, and speech-language pathology should look like and how that therapy should be documented. When reviewing regulatory language, it is interesting to note that providing a definition is often deferred to the disciplines themselves. Over time, when concerns arise about clarity, payer sources then begin to try to drive documentation expectations that derive from the respective professions themselves. As an example, refinements to the Home Health PPS have contained additional detail asking for tests and measures to be present in therapy assessments.

Looking at therapy educational curriculums, it becomes clear that the utilization of tests and measures is a long-standing expectation for all three disciplines and is not an expectation created by Medicare or specific to home health. There is also no mention in Home Health PPS of any specific tests and measures to be used because it is up to the skilled therapist to assess his or her patient base and choose tools that are appropriate, meaningful, and relevant. Many home health therapists are waiting for Medicare to create the list of recommended tests or to decide which measure is "approved." Therapists are not in a position to do that nor should they even try. Therapists need to take a long look at their own discipline and define as a group what constitutes skilled care as well as the documentation content that best supports the medical necessity and addresses interventions as well as progress.

OASIS: Impact on Therapy Practice

The topic of therapy documentation in home health cannot overlook the both the role and influence of the Outcome and Assessment Information Set (OASIS). The acronym itself no longer invokes images of warm sandy beaches with swaying palm trees and a gorgeous sunset for any clinician who has worked in the home health setting for any period of time. Very few, if any, clinicians will volunteer to complete this document and some have become quite good at avoiding it. The general consensus of many is that the tool is "extra" work and completed for the benefit of Medicare with little to no direct use to the clinician trying to care for people in need. A critical element of home health since the year 2000, OASIS remains an object of frustration and confusion and, in many ways, disconnected from therapy documentation.

Data Collection

Prior to the year 2000, there was no consistent outcome data specific to home health. Agencies created their own tools for issues they felt were important, like patient satisfaction, but there was no mechanism by which one agency could compare its performance against another agency or against state or national reference information. Medicare, the largest payer source for skilled home health services, grew more and more concerned that there was nothing to quantify the impact of the care being provided.

The need to create a standardized tool that would collect the same information about patients seen by home health providers in Maine, California, North Dakota, or Louisiana became clear. Many people were involved in the development of the items and responses, and the end result was a data collection tool that was, and is, discipline neutral. That being said, each discipline brings a different set of expertise to the data collection and can have different reactions to and levels of comfort with the individual items. This has led to the idea that there are "therapy" OASIS items—namely, the functional areas such as ambulation, transfers, and bathing. As therapists, a certain level of skill in these areas is a natural extension of what they would "typically" look at when assessing patients, but that does not make data collection in these areas limited to only therapists.

OASIS items regarding wounds, dyspnea, and incontinence have, at times, been thought of as "nursing" questions but, in reality, are within the scope of a therapist to collect information about. The overriding theme of OASIS is to collect accurate information about a patient in order to determine what changes have occurred over time as a result of specific interventions—which is the core of delivering high-quality care in any setting. Every discipline involved in home health has a stake in showing positive patient outcomes.

Determining Impact of Care

The ability to show the impact of care begins with an accurate assessment at the beginning of the episode. According to the Medicare *Conditions of Participation* (§484.55), "a registered nurse must conduct an initial assessment visit to determine the immediate care and support needs of the patient; and, for Medicare patients, to determine eligibility for the Medicare home health benefit, including homebound status." In cases that include nursing and therapy services, the registered nurse is required to complete the admission visit regardless of patient diagnosis or staffing availability. The *Conditions of Participation* (§484.55) continues, adding, "when rehabilitation therapy service (speech language pathology, physical therapy, or occupational therapy) is the only service ordered by the physician, and if the need for that service establishes program eligibility, the initial assessment visit may be made by the appropriate rehabilitation skilled professional."

For Medicare patients, the initial assessment, inclusive of OASIS, can be done by the physical therapist or the speech-language pathologist when there are no nursing orders present. The need for occupational therapy alone does not meet the criteria of a qualifying service and means that an occupational therapist is not able to admit a Medicare patient to home health. They may be able to do so with other payer sources, so each one should be verified independently with respect to coverage criteria.

Completion of a discharge, transfer, resumption of care, or recertification OASIS can be done by nursing and any of the three therapies, and there is no hierarchy of which one can do it. Therapist assistants are not able to complete the document itself but can provide valuable insights in to the patient's abilities when they understand the importance of the tool.

Therapists and the Start of Care Assessment

There has been discussion and debate about the ability of a therapist to complete a start of care assessment. There are components of this task such as the drug regimen review, skin assessment, and incontinence that some deem as not actual "therapy." Although by definition these areas are not traditionally seen as a therapy task in home health, this unique setting challenges therapists to understand they are treating entire patients and not isolated joints or specific problems in a vacuum.

In the hospital setting, there is a call light option to summon a nurse quickly to the bedside when needed. In the home, a nurse can be accessible over the phone but may not reach the home for a period of time or it may be a case where no nursing services have been ordered. Therapists must keep in mind that what is actually being done is a screening of the patient to determine if and when other services are warranted and if this is within the scope of a therapist. It is understandable when an agency makes the decision to not have therapists completing admissions based on limited staff availability, but it is concerning when the decision is made based on a perception that therapists are not capable of completing that level of assessment.

Therapists must be clear as to the difference between a true scope of practice issue and a task that a specific therapist is not comfortable and/or competent to complete. Scope of practice is defined by regulation whereas personal competence is a result of training and experience. Consider this example: Would it be legal for a licensed nurse in your state to draw blood? In the legal sense it would be accepted practice. Would you allow any random licensed nurse in your state to draw blood from you? You would probably not allow that. You would want a nurse that is capable and knows how to draw blood well based on level of experience. The same logic applies to some of the tasks OASIS requires a therapist to do. Can a licensed therapist conduct a thorough skin assessment in your state? It is within the scope of practice. Are you as a therapist comfortable and competent completing a skin assessment? If not, the issue becomes how you will go about gaining knowledge and practice. With any of these areas, it is the responsibility of the professional to know what the specific details are in the scope of practice document for the state in which he or she practices to ensure that expectations are within the scope of each discipline.

Drug Regimen Review

Taking on an even more volatile issue in home health therapy is the drug regimen review. It appears that the visceral reaction of some to this issue is complicated by a certain level of misunderstanding. Therapists tend to be quite territorial and protective of their patients. They firmly believe that if they assess for something, they become responsible for seeing that issue is taken care of. Applying that to medication management, being asked to look over the medication profile does not mean the therapist has to directly address any issues that are found. Specific to physical therapy, Medicare has commented on "Medication management and education: Physical therapists are more than capable of completing the drug regimen review item. It is within the scope of the physical therapist to perform a patient screen in which medication issues are assessed even if the physical therapist does not perform the specific care needed to address the medication issue." It is important to focus on the word choice of "patient screen" because it puts this issue into perspective and reflects that the purpose is to know if there are problems and to bring in the appropriate services to effectively address them.

Collaboration for Improved Accuracy

Agencies must abide by regulations in order participate in the Medicare program as well as any state or local regulations that apply. It is important to understand that OASIS is a document with a single signature attesting to the accuracy of the information collected. Combining the home health regulations with the OASIS requirements has led to the strong perception that the OASIS is the responsibility of one clinician alone. The *OASIS-C Guidance Manual* confirms that, on admission, there is a five-day window in which the clinician is able to collect information about the patient. This is the opportunity for all members of the care team involved with the patient to collaborate in order to ensure the highest possible level of data accuracy. It also becomes clear that participation in OASIS data collection is the responsibility of the interdisciplinary team regardless of actual document completion. The typical length of time spent in the home with the patient on an admission visit ranges from an hour and a half to two hours. Even the most experienced home health clinician, regardless of discipline, can have challenges that impact the assessment. Consider the following two admission situations:

* Mrs. Evans is a 70-year-old woman referred to home health after an exacerbation of her heart failure that resulted in a hospital admission lasting three weeks. Prior to the visit, an extensive packet of information was given to the clinician assigned to admit her. In the home, the clinician encounters a patient who is very open about her concerns regarding her health situation and her ability to continue to care for herself at home. She reports needing help with dressing, bathing, and will not walk alone due to her fear of falling. The patient's daughter is present during the visit and confirms what the patient is reporting based on extensive knowledge of her history and observing her self-care abilities since returning home.

* Mr. Williams is a 95-year-old man who lives alone. His wife died several years ago, and his family lives out of the area and sees him infrequently. He was discharged from the nursing home after a recent mild stroke. The only information the clinician has ahead of the admission visit was the diagnosis of cerebrovascular accident and his demographic details. During the visit, the patient repeatedly insists he is "fine" and "does not need help." He reports he is able to dress, bathe, and prepare meals on his own and takes his medication regularly. The clinician tries to call the daughter-in-law to confirm the information without response.

Envision the clinician trying to gather assessment information about Mrs. Evans compared to Mr. Williams. The expectation that a clinician can collect completely accurate information about every single patient in an hour and a half to two hours may not be realistic.

The majority of agencies have a review process for the OASIS document to ensure data collection is accurate. There may be an entire department of people who spend their days reading OASIS documentation. Clinicians have learned to be apprehensive of these staff members because a call from them means something was wrong and has to be corrected. Busy clinicians may become so overwhelmed with corrections that they no longer actually care about an accurate response and simply want to know which responses will make the reviewer happy. When clinicians show a pattern of inaccuracy, many agencies will put them back into additional OASIS training—spending a considerable amount of resources, both time and financial, repeatedly trying to help clinicians to "get it." Since the year 2000, this has been an all too familiar cycle in many home health agencies as they try to manage OASIS. There is another option to consider: collaboration between clinicians who have seen the patient within the first five days since the start of care.

Returning to Mr. Williams and the limited information the admitting clinician had to start with and could reasonably get from the patient, the occupational therapist came out the day after the admission visit to complete her initial assessment. As it turns out, she has worked with him before and discharged him about six months ago. She recalls he had some significant cognitive issues and was not consistent with taking his medications. He was bathing on his own when she discharged him but currently his balance and general fatigue would mean he could not safely complete that task alone at this time. The occupational therapist clearly documents this in her assessment *but* does not attempt to look at the OASIS responses in these areas or communicate specifically to the admitting clinician other than reporting the planned frequency and duration for activities of daily living (ADL) retraining. When the reviewer in the office looks at the OASIS and the occupational therapy evaluation side by side, she notices the differences and cannot figure out why the admitting clinician "missed" this information and calls her to ask her to change the responses.

Would it not be better for the occupational therapist and the admitting clinician to collaborate before the OASIS is submitted to create consistent information? No one is suggesting that the five-day window should be used in every case. For our Mrs. Evans, there was a lot of good information collected on the admission visit and an accurate OASIS could be generated from that without waiting for additional insights. In addition, the five-day window is *not* about how long a clinician has to completely fill out the tool. It is about having the opportunity to go back and conduct additional data collection as the admitting clinician or to seek out insights from others. Note the use of the term *collaboration*—it is not acceptable practice to carve the OASIS tool into parts and have different disciplines complete sections independent of each other. Many of the frustrations with OASIS data collection are rooted in the larger issues facing home health—collaboration, communication, and documentation.

Incorporating OASIS Into Therapy Documentation

OASIS influence should extend beyond the completion of the actual tool. There are many important pieces of information that are relevant on all assessments of a patient. With nursing services doing the majority of home health admissions in many agencies, the initial contact a nurse has with a patient more often than not involves OASIS as part of the comprehensive assessment.

In light of the fact that occupational therapists are not completing admissions to home health for Medicare patients, these evaluations can be disconnected from OASIS and appear very discipline-specific, which leaves important broader issues undocumented—like the presence of incontinence or a current pressure ulcer. Although speech pathologists are able to admit Medicare patients, the limitations related to staffing issues in many agencies limits this practice. For physical therapists, there are a significant number of patients being admitted by this service, and these assessments include not only the discipline-specific information but also address additional issues by virtue of OASIS.

When looking at the physical therapy evaluation done after a nursing admission, it appears that there is almost a split personality at work. When admitting a patient, the physical therapist will note issues with dyspnea and interfering pain, but these are often absent on an evaluation. Why would those same issues not be relevant regardless of the formal inclusion of the OASIS document? In light of the continued concerns raised by Medicare as to the medical necessity of skilled therapy services, the disconnect present in many documentation tools and content creates a significant opportunity to link what therapists "typically" do with larger measurements of home health quality.

Home Health Compare

When looking at the Home Health Compare outcome scores, accessible to anyone at *www.medicare.gov*, it can be tempting to gravitate toward some more than others.

+ Improvement in ambulation/locomotion

+ Improvement in bathing

- Improvement of oral medications

- Improvement in transferring

- Improvement with pain interfering with activity

- Any emergent care provided

- Acute care hospitalizations

- Improvement in dyspnea

- Improvement in urinary incontinence

- Discharge to the community

- Improvement in the status of surgical wounds

- Emergent care wound infections/deteriorating wound status

The outcome relating to ambulation appears to be physical therapy, bathing would be occupational therapy, and oral medication would be nursing. There is a flaw in this plan because not every home health patient receives nursing and not every home health patient receives therapy. Based on utilization, it is not possible to hold one specific discipline responsible for one specific outcome. The team approach is a key element to effective care delivery that creates solid documentation as an end product. OASIS items collect data elements, but they do not answer the question of why a problem exists. That is left to clinical judgment, which then triggers which discipline or mix of disciplines is the most effective and efficient plan for each individual patient.

Since 2000, agencies have been challenged to embrace the idea of interfering pain. Healthcare providers are very familiar and comfortable with using the zero to 10 pain scale in all settings. Patients are so used to being asked about this that they may even greet the therapist arriving at the home with "I am a five today" without even being asked. Level of pain is an important component of the assessment, but the outcome measure related to pain is *not* tied to or driven by a number. It is a noble goal to decrease a patient's pain level in every case, but that may not be realistic given the population serviced by home health.

The Home Health Compare outcome is measured by the following OASIS item:

OASIS (M1242) Frequency of pain interfering with patient's activity or movement:

- ❑ 0 - Patient has no pain

- ❑ 1 - Patient has pain that does not interfere with activity or movement

- ❑ 2 - Less often than daily

- ❑ 3 - Daily, but not constantly

- ❑ 4 - All of the time

As can be seen in the item, there is no mention of a pain level but the focus is on how the pain, regardless of level, is interfering with the patient from a functionality and quality of life perspective. Is it possible that a patient would rate her pain as "0" because she is sitting still and has just taken her medications? Pressing further, it is determined that pain is worse in the morning and makes dressing a much harder task. The score for M1242 would be response 3 despite a current pain level being reported as "0."

As we work with this patient and provide occupational therapy to address the dressing issues, we can impact how pain is affecting her life. At discharge, she reports much less difficulty with dressing so her M1242 score would show improvement compared to the admission score. During the discharge visit, she reports a pain level of 2 and the therapist may feel the need to panic. It appears she is "worse" because her pain level went up, but the outcome being pursued is pain management in the functional and quality of life areas. If the pain level is lower at discharge that is a good thing but not the measurement of the outcome "improvement in pain." Here is the gap: does a therapist only think along these lines when completing an OASIS but not on a therapy evaluation? The overwhelming majority of therapy evaluation tools collect information about level of pain, what makes it worse, what makes it better, and so on. What is missing is the link between pain and interference. With therapy being obviously tied to function, the impact of pain on these tasks should be evident in the documentation and consistent with the OASIS responses.

Along similar lines to interfering pain is the issue of dyspnea. OASIS data collection in this area is not directly tied to any specific pulmonary diagnosis. Think about a time when you have had a bad cold or flu and been in bed for several days. When you start to feel better, the stairs in your home can seem like a mountain and climbing up them results in shortness of breath. This is not necessarily indicative of acquiring a pulmonary disease but a by-product of inactivity due to illness. The OASIS item is asking for the level of activity that is provoking the shortness of breath.

OASIS (M1400) When is the patient dyspneic or noticeably short of breath?

- ❑   0 - Patient is not short of breath

- ❑   1 - When walking more than 20 feet, climbing stairs

- ❑   2 - With moderate exertion (e.g., while dressing, using commode or bedpan, walking distances less than 20 feet)

- ❑   3 - With minimal exertion (e.g., while eating, talking, or performing other ADLs) or with agitation

- ❑   4 - At rest (during day or night)

Agencies have spent a significant amount of time educating clinicians who complete admissions on this particular item with the end result being many admissions reporting that the patient is a response 2, with moderate exertion. Within days of the admission visit by nursing, the physical therapist completes an evaluation that includes information that the patient is ambulating 50 feet with standby assistance and a walker but no mention at all about shortness of breath. It is possible that the patient did not present with dyspnea on the therapy evaluation but it is also possible that the therapist was not thinking about and ultimately documenting these findings as part of a complete assessment. For occupational therapy, awareness of dyspnea as a component of assessing dressing and other self-care tasks is a key element. Shortness of breath while speaking, if present, should show up as part of the speech-language pathology evaluation.

Therapists must also consider issues the patient may have that can complicate the plan of care. The cognitive behavioral section of OASIS has often been artificially connected to patient diagnosis. As an example, a patient diagnosed with dementia is more likely to have scores reflecting issues with memory or confusion whereas the patient who does not have a diagnosis along those lines is scored as not having any issues. Consider the following OASIS item:

OASIS (M1700) Cognitive Functioning: Patient's current (day of assessment) level of alertness, orientation, comprehension, concentration, and immediate memory for simple commands:

- ❑   0 - Alert/oriented, able to focus and shift attention, comprehends and recalls task directions independently

- ❑   1 - Requires prompting (cuing, repetition, reminders) only under stressful or unfamiliar conditions

- ❑   2 - Requires assistance and some direction in specific situations (e.g., on all tasks involving shifting of attention), or consistently requires low stimulus environment due to distractibility

- ❑   3 - Requires considerable assistance in routine situations; is not alert and oriented or is unable to shift attention and recall directions more than half the time

- ❑   4 - Totally dependent due to disturbances such as constant disorientation, coma, persistent vegetative state, or delirium

Notice that there is no mention of a diagnosis but a focus on the current level of alertness *and* orientation, comprehension, concentration, and immediate memory for simple commands. Review of records indicates that clinicians may only be reading as far as response "0," while not looking at the rest of that response that addressed attention, comprehension, and recall. In reality, many patients are fine with information they already knew but the introduction of teaching about wound care or a home program may be a different situation. The clinician needs to understand that by selecting response 0, Medicare is being told that the patient can also recall task directions independently. If that is true, consider how much repeat training the patient would actually require. If true, consider how the medical necessity of repeat visits of teaching would be supported. This is not to say that no home health patients should be scored as "0," but clinicians need to think about the fact that if repeated teaching of new information will be required, maybe the response of "1" would be more appropriate. Moving to the therapy documentation specifically, issues of memory, attention, and recall are far too often either absent or appear to be fine. The amount of questions related to cognitive behavioral issues in OASIS indicate that Medicare is looking for information reflecting the complexity of the patients being served, and this level of detail will provide additional support for skilled care.

Management of oral medications raises issues previously touched upon with respect to scope of practice, but it is imperative to really understand the OASIS items and responses involved in determining improvement in this area.

(M2020) Management of Oral Medications: Patient's current ability to prepare and take all oral medications reliably and safely, including administration of the correct dosage at the appropriate times/intervals. Excludes injectable and IV medications. (NOTE: This refers to ability, not compliance or willingness.)

☐   0 - Able to independently take the correct oral medication(s) and proper dosage(s) at the correct times

☐   1 - Able to take medication(s) at the correct times if:

    (a) Individual dosages are prepared in advance by another person; *or*

    (b) Another person develops a drug diary or chart

☐   2 - Able to take medication(s) at the correct times if given reminders by another person at the appropriate times

☐   3 - Unable to take medication unless administered by another person

☐   N/A - No oral medications prescribed

There is no mention in the item of the patient being able to recite his entire medication list by memory including the chemical composition of each. Limited knowledge of the proper medication regimen may be a contributing factor impacting oral medication management, but one cannot overlook the functionality of this item. When assessing gait, has the physical therapist asked the patient where she keeps her medications? If they are in the bathroom upstairs and the patient has to take them three times per day, is she safely able to access them or would assistance be necessary? Occupational therapy is closely tied to fine motor skills, and these are clearly relevant to the act of opening pill bottles. Should the occupational therapy evaluation show routine assessment of this task as it can have a significant impact on patient safety and hospitalization risks? The speech therapy evaluation may highlight issues with memory or problem solving, but how does that impact medication management? All three therapies have the potential to have a positive impact on this specific outcome depending on why the issue exists, yet little information about this is clearly documented by any of them as part of the assessment or the plan of care.

Home health has been directed by Medicare to be an active participant in reducing rehospitalization rates, and that is reflected in the outcome measure specific to this issue. There is an OASIS item that should be considered part of an agency's efforts to decrease the rate. It also represents the challenge of interdisciplinary care management.

OASIS (M1032) Risk for Hospitalization: Which of the following signs or symptoms characterize this patient as at risk for hospitalization? (Mark all that apply.)

- ❑ 1 - Recent decline in mental, emotional, or behavioral status

- ❑ 2 - Multiple hospitalizations (two or more) in the past 12 months

- ❑ 3 - History of falls (two or more falls—or any fall with an injury—in the past year)

- ❑ 4 - Taking five or more medications

- ❑ 5 - Frailty indicators (e.g., weight loss, self-reported exhaustion)

- ❑ 6 - Other

- ❑ 7 - None of the above

This information is collected at the start of care by the admitting clinician. Once complete, it will be subject to the review process and then transmitted to Medicare. If an agency is truly working on decreasing preventable hospitalizations, having this information available only to the clinician who did the admission and the review staff would not be the best use of this data. Capturing risks should translate into a plan of care to address these individually for each patient and trigger the inclusion of other services to assist as indicated. Some will say that they have challenges accessing this information or they do not even know for sure who did the admission. This item and the follow-up it implies embody interdisciplinary patient-focused care and highlight the primary roadblocks many agencies and clinicians struggle with—communication, collaboration, and documentation.

Connecting OASIS to Therapy

No one is suggesting that therapists in home health will love the OASIS and jump at the opportunity to be involved in data collection. Several items were discussed in this chapter, but the same level of consideration and discussion should happen with the OASIS data overall to maximize the ability to integrate it into care planning for all providers, including the therapy assistants. It is a unique tool that requires both baseline and ongoing training and must move from the perception of "extra work" to an integral part of patient-centered care delivery. The tool provides insight to therapy as to larger outcome measurement issues for which they are uniquely qualified to address. Being an active participant in collecting accurate data and showing consistency in discipline-specific documentation will better support the medical necessity and inclusion of therapy services in the plan of care designed to meet the needs of each individual patient.

Assessments: The Foundation for Medical Necessity

Building a therapy plan of care is similar to building a house. The foundation sets the tone for the overall quality of the building, and if the condition of the materials is not up to code, it will not support the ultimate structure. The ability to create a solid foundation requires training, experience, and good decision-making. The initial visit with a patient is the opportunity to create the baseline upon which additional visits can be supported as medically necessary. Before diving in to more specifics, it is important to start with the proper focus.

Think back to your first day of therapy school—how much did you know? If you were like most of your classmates, you were more concerned with finding the right room and choosing a good seat than having any specific clinical expertise. Time was then spent learning assessment skills from books and lectures, and practicing on other students, friends, and family members.

Along came the clinical rotations and the opportunity to practice these newfound assessment skills on real patients. How much did you really know even then? At the time, the laboratory jacket and name badge conveyed a certain level of competence that might have been more than you really felt you possessed. Those early assessments usually involved some sort of "cheat sheet" or list of key items you did not want to forget, carefully kept in an easy-to-reach pocket or attached to a clipboard. You became brave and empowered at some point and tried doing an assessment without looking at that sheet. What happened? As with any new therapist, you probably missed a few things and had the uncomfortable pleasure of going back to the patient to finish the task. Once out of school, you gained expertise and confidence, and it is doubtful that you carry any sort of assessment cheat sheet anymore. And now, you are currently utilizing your therapy assessment skills on other human beings without even thinking about it.

During your most recent trip to the local mall, did you notice things about complete strangers? An odd gait pattern, the walker being carried and not really on the floor, or a fellow diner coughing regularly after sipping her drink may have caught your attention as your therapy radar scans the surroundings. You realize that you are now a therapist 24/7 and are actually unable to shut that part of you off. Even family gatherings trigger the questions, "Can you look at my hip?" and "My shoulder is sore. Can I have a massage?" while you are trying to relax and enjoy time together.

Your current level of skill is wonderful for you and your patients, but it can be quite problematic for your documentation. Much of a therapy assessment is now more instinct than specific thoughts, and this has led to documentation that far too often is limited in detail and creates the impression that the skills of a therapist were not required to achieve the same level of content. At the core, this is why therapy documentation issues in most cases are very correctable when focus is restored, starting with the initial assessment. Move away from the obligatory, "If you didn't document it, you didn't do it" to a mind-set of displaying your clinical skills and getting credit for how hard it was to gain the level of expertise you currently possess.

Homebound Status

To qualify for home-based services to be paid for under the Medicare benefit, the patient has to be "homebound." It is required to determine homebound status at the time of the admission assessment and periodically over the course of care. This task is not limited exclusively to the discipline that completed the start of care visit because it is the responsibility of all clinicians to confirm that the patient qualifies for services throughout the 60-day episode. Homebound status has been a challenge to define clearly in the minds of even the most seasoned home health clinicians. Orientation for some therapists has included variations of the directive to never document the patient walked on grass because that would mean he or she went outside. Being homebound does not mean confined to bed nor does it imply that the patient is a home hostage. Discharge is not suddenly mandatory the minute the patient crosses the threshold and steps outside. The regulations themselves do not have a list of approved places and acceptable durations of time the patient can be out of the home. There are three main components to homebound status that should be considered simultaneously, and none of them are tied to the destination.

ASSESSMENTS: THE FOUNDATION FOR MEDICAL NECESSITY

1. **Infrequent.** The patient is allowed to be away from the home periodically. This is because if a patient is able to leave the home regularly for other activities, then he or she should be capable of accessing medical care—therapy, nursing, or social work—on an outpatient basis. When that is the case, he or she no longer qualifies for services to come to the home. There is no number in the regulations so frequency must be discussed with the patient over the course of care, and when the interdisciplinary team confirms regularity of leaving the home, discharge should be considered.

2. **Short duration.** The time the patient is actually out of the home should not be for hours on end and occurring routinely (see "infrequent"). This ties once again to the purpose of a home health benefit as it is designed for people who cannot access necessary medical care outside the home. There is no specified length of time that is confirmed as the acceptable range, so clinicians need to assess each individual patient and determine what his or her status may be in this area.

3. **Taxing effort.** This is probably the largest confirming aspect of homebound status. It speaks to the fact that the physical demands, psychosocial issues, and/or safety concerns are high enough that they limit the ability of the patient to receive necessary medical care outside of the home. Here are some examples:

    a. Mr. Anderson is unable to walk more than 30 feet with his walker before he becomes very short of breath and must sit to rest. His ability to participate effectively in outpatient therapy is insufficient at this time as he fatigues quickly.

    b. Mrs. Greyhound has pain in both her hips and requires her daughter's assistance to dress and bathe. Her pain becomes intolerable when riding in a car for more than 10 minutes, and she is more than 30 minutes away from her physician's office. She is new to warfarin and requires regular laboratory draws as well as significant monitoring and education but cannot get to her doctor to have these needs met at this time.

    c. Mr. Peterson has issues with anxiety and when he keeps his regular routine he is able to function fairly well without major incidents. He fell at home about a month ago and needs follow-up on lower extremity biomechanics but the initial attempts at outpatient physical therapy were unsuccessful as they made him so upset he could not participate.

To be clear on the homebound issue, a patient cannot simply decide he or she wants to stay home and receive care in a way that is more convenient. If that were true, nearly everyone in the country would make that choice from time to time and enjoy the respite. The Medicare benefit is not based on personal preferences but on the needs of the patient. In the examples provided, it can be seen that there are a variety of issues that can cause a person to be homebound and support why it takes the clinical decision-making skills of a nurse or therapist to determine the appropriate level of care a patient requires.

Medicare has been asked to provide clarity to the homebound issue, and the end result has been a list of examples. Example is the key word because the examples do not serve as a checklist of "approved" locations or activities. The patient is allowed to leave the home for medically related appointments, attend church services, get his or her hair done (a very positive event for many home health patients—especially the females), go for a walk around the block, or participate in family events such as birthdays, weddings, holidays, and funerals. Keep in mind that homebound status is not tied to any specific destination and must be confirmed based on frequency of leaving the home, the duration of the absences, and the amount of effort to complete the activity.

Here are some examples to consider:

1. Mrs. Matthews is a Medicare recipient and has orders for home health. This past week she went to get her hair done and stopped to visit with her friend for her recent birthday. She went to church and had her routine physician appointment as well. She completed all of these tasks with few problems and her daughter drove her to all these locations as she has not driven in the past five years. Mrs. Matthews would not meet the homebound criteria despite all of those activities being on the example list from Medicare. She is leaving the home regularly, gone for varying amounts of time, and does not require significant effort.

2. Mr. Patten is a Medicare recipient and has orders for home health. Yesterday he went to the grocery store with his son, a task he does once or twice a month as it involves picking up his medications and he likes to talk about them with the pharmacist. On this recent trip, he was able to walk into the store but became very fatigued. The son secured one of the scooters from the store but Mr. Patten was unable to maneuver it safely due to pain in his hands and some newly emerging cognitive issues. He ended up waiting in the car as his son bought the necessary items. Once

home, Mr. Patten went to take a nap and later complained of increased pain in both hands and his legs that is still present today despite taking his pain medications correctly. Mr. Patten would be considered homebound even though grocery shopping is not mentioned on the Medicare list of examples. He leaves infrequently and clearly there are taxing effort issues that make it unrealistic for him to access medical care on an outpatient basis at this time to address his needs.

The determination and confirmation of homebound status is a key component of assessments as well as routine visits for all three therapy disciplines. Careful consideration of what makes leaving the home a "taxing effort" should be an integral part of the documentation. It is also important to keep homebound status in its proper place as it is a key aspect of the Medicare coverage criteria but it is not the goal of home health providers to keep them at that level. Think about how a patient is introduced to the concept of homebound status. It occurs on the admission visit, which many will report is routinely an hour and a half to two hours of time with the patient.

Amidst all the questions being asked, papers being signed, and tasks being demonstrated, the patient is basically read the Miranda rights of home health—if the patient gets better and can leave the home, the agency will discharge. This message is delivered on the very first interaction with the agency and sets the stage that progress is not necessarily a good thing in the eyes of the patient. They are probably at their sickest point when services begin and are told that recovery will mean loss of services. For some patients this is not an issue as they are more than motivated to not need services for longer than they have to. Others appreciate the care so much that they do not want it to end for quite some time. Home health therapists can get caught in this idea as well and miss the true purpose of providing skilled care. It is to improve the patient's situation so that they are no longer homebound.

Think about the patient who is being prepared for ultimate discharge to outpatient therapy services. In order to participate effectively in the outpatient setting, the patient has to get out of bed, get cleaned up and dressed, take the necessary medications, eat a meal, be transported to the outpatient center, participate in one to three hours of therapy (depending on the services ordered in the plan of care), then be transported home and be a functional human being the rest of the day. There are so many components to the process that active busy clinicians may not even think of. Will a patient be properly prepared if the occupational therapist comes out on Monday to work on dressing in the morning, speech-language pathologist comes out Monday afternoon to help problem solve safe medication management, and the physical therapist comes out on Tuesday and walks the patient to the car door and back? The necessary tasks were not assessed in the functional order they would naturally occur in but were artificially spread over two calendar days.

There have been questions raised about the level of ability a person needs to have to function in the community. In the *Journal of Geriatric Physical Therapy* (Volume 33, Number 2, April/June 2010, pp. 56–63), there is an article entitled "Defining community ambulation from the perspective of the older adult." Based on that article, the following list of questions has been put together to provoke thoughts about how care is being planned for the home health patients and consideration for how they may want to function after discharge from services:

Can the patient:

+ Carry a 5-pound weight for more than 1,000 feet?

+ Carry packages averaging 6 to 7 pounds for short distances?

+ Walk a minimum of 1,000 feet per errand for two to three errands per trip?

+ Change speeds and maintain balance?

+ Negotiate safely around obstacles, slopes, or curbs while looking in a variety of directions?

+ Multitask while walking (walk and talk, walk and look from side to side or up and down)?

+ Carry a package up and down the stairs?

+ Safely engage in postural transitions such as changing directions, reaching, looking up or down or sideways, moving backward?

+ Rise from a chair without the use of arms with minimal effort?

+ Walk at 4 feet per second for at least one minute to cross a street?

+ Walk at a minimum speed of 160 feet per minute, or about 2.6 feet per second?

These questions help to set the appropriate stage for the initial assessment of patients in this unique setting. Therapists in home health need a solid understanding of homebound status and need to make it a key element of a thorough assessment as well as determining a course of care. This is more than picking a particular predetermined check box response because it requires a skill set that then connects specific findings to the reason or reasons a patient should receive services under the Medicare home health benefit.

Initiating the Assessment

The gathering of information about a patient begins over the phone during the initial contact to set up an appointment. The therapy radar goes off when patients do not remember being in the nursing home last week, cannot hear well so that volume has to be increased, or repeat statements or questions several times over the course of the conversation. Once the door opens for the first visit, data collection begins immediately and topics are seen simultaneously. As clinical expertise has increased, the ability to assess the physical ability, cognitive status, visual challenges, and the environmental concerns while interacting with a patient has grown and developed.

Part of the drive to become a therapist is the desire to help people, but this instinct must be kept in check during an assessment. By its very nature, the assessment process is designed to collect information about what is the current situation of the patient without any influence of the therapist. Routinely seen as problem solvers, intervention can be provided without even thinking about it, and when documentation occurs after that point the assessment may no longer be accurate and clearly in support of the need for skilled care. For example, while assessing Mr. Jasper's ability to get on and off the toilet, the therapist sees that he is struggling to complete the task safely. The toilet is much too low for him, and he is trying to push himself up with the toilet paper hanger and the vanity. The therapist noticed the bedside commode frame in the dining room and asks Mr. Jasper if it is okay to show him how to use the frame over the toilet. He agrees. Once in place, he attempts the transfer again and is now about to complete the task safely and independently and is very pleased with this. Later that day, the therapist is completing the assessment note and for toilet transfers documents Mr. Jasper's ability as "independent with a commode frame in place" but is this correct? His actual ability when assessed was the assistance and safety concerns noted upon arrival to the home, not after a skilled intervention was provided. The instruction and relocation of the commode frame would still be documented but in a different area of the visit. If the level of ability is, in fact, documented as independent, the intervention and skill of the therapist specific to that task is lost. Timing of completion of the documentation as well as clarity on what defines the patient's true ability are factors that can enhance or detract from medical necessity.

Prior level of function

Regardless of the assessment being completed by the physical therapist, occupational therapist, or the speech-language pathologist, there is one area that is clearly required to be present. It is the documentation of the patient's prior level of function (PLOF). The inclusion of this information is not a home health–specific idea or something dreamed up by Medicare and other payers. Therapists are taught this concept very early on in training but, somewhere along the line, have let the detail slide or become absent completely. Agencies are reporting that when attempts are being made to appeal a denial for payment of therapy services rendered, PLOF is being looked at closely, especially at the level of the administrative law judge. Absence of this information does not strengthen the case for skilled therapy but raises the concern about how much improvement was realistically expected when a baseline level with time frames is not documented.

Some therapists comment that the reason they do not document on PLOF involves two issues. The first is that they were not there to confirm what the patient and/or caregiver are reporting so they are unsure if is accurate. The second is a concern that if their interventions improve a patient beyond the documented PLOF, then they will be at risk for payment denial. As to the accuracy of self-reported information, this is a risk for both prior and current functional abilities but does not remove the importance of it. It is understood that the details are not based on direct observation of the therapist, and if there are questions as to accuracy, this can be documented as part of the information by the therapist. As to the second issue, it is entirely possible that the interventions can help the patient attain a higher than expected level of functional ability, especially if there were little or no interventions for a considerable length of time. Once again, this does not make documentation of the PLOF optional as goals can be updated and should be supported in the medical record to indicate why skilled care would continue to be effective. PLOF provides a general context for performance and a baseline expectation to support the necessity of therapy interventions.

Compare these two patients:

1. Mr. Adams is 70 years old and fell out of bed, fracturing his left hip. He was taken to the emergency room and admitted later that day for a hip pinning. Prior to this fall, he was taking daily walks with no assistive device around the assisted living facility in which he resides and routinely participated in community outings. He currently can only walk about 5 feet with his walker and has considerable pain as well as substantial issues with maintaining his weight-bearing restriction. The physical therapy gait goal is 300 feet with a cane independently.

2. Mr. Jones is 70 years old and fell out of bed, fracturing his left hip. He was taken to the emergency room and admitted later that day for a hip pinning. Prior to this fall he required minimal assistance to transfer from his bed to a scooter, which was his primary method of mobility for the past five years due to severe arthritis. Other than taking a few steps as part of the transfer process, he has not been a functional ambulator. He currently requires moderate assistance to complete transfers safely. The physical therapy gait goal is 300 feet with a cane independently.

It was intentional to make the patients' ages, injuries, and surgical follow-up the same. PLOF clearly created two different expectations as to what level of activity could reasonably be expected for each of them. When the goals for physical therapy are the same in both cases, the first appears appropriate while the second does not.

Use of "independent"

When completing assessments, there is an entire continuum of terminology available to therapists. It ranges from dependence to independence with a variety of levels in between. In order to effectively communicate the status of the patient, care must be taken in choosing the most appropriate description. Inconsistencies between therapists can lead to confusion for third-party reviewers. When therapists have worked together for some time they can become quite comfortable that they are all speaking the same language only to have a record denied payment over lack of medical necessity. Clear understanding of the levels of assistance should be periodically reevaluated to ensure all therapists are applying them in a similar and appropriate fashion.

One specific term has been a contributing factor to confusion regarding the need for therapy services: independent. At first glance, it can be hard to see why this word would be an issue as it appears straightforward. It simply means the patient is able to consistently complete a given task without assistance of any kind whenever he or she would choose to do it without safety concerns. Being independent directly implies that there is no need for skilled intervention in this particular area. Although therapists may believe that this term is being used correctly in assessment documentation, here are examples from real records:

+ "Independent but unsafe"

+ "Independent but unsteady"

+ "Independent with supervision"

+ "Independent but requires repeated attempts"

+ "Independent with verbal cues"

There is no place in therapy documentation for "independent but . . ." or combining independent with other levels of assistance such as supervision and verbal cues. A patient is either independent or not, there is no half way. Some will argue that this is "not what I meant," but it is easy to see why a payer source would deny payment for interventions to address activities that the patient is already capable of performing. Connected to this discussion is the term "modified independent" which has found its way into home health documentation.

Functional independence measure tool

Therapists who have practiced in a rehabilitation unit are familiar with the Functional Independence Measure tool. Now referred to simply as FIM™, it is a proprietary tool specific to inpatient rehabilitation and requires permission and training to use. Modified independent is a level of assistance defined by and attached to this one tool and outside of it does not have a clear and consistent meaning. Therapists will insist they know what they meant and often report it is "independent with equipment."

Due to the lack of a meaningful definition outside of inpatient rehabilitation, it is strongly recommended that the designation not be used in home health. Record review often reflects this term being applied and then additional interventions being provided. Bottom line, if the patient is already "independent" with modification or none, there is no need for the therapist to continue to address this issue. Independence is the highest level of function. There is no "super independent" level to attain. Think through this example:

On the initial assessment visit, the occupational therapist documents that Mrs. Kelly is able to bathe at a level of modified independent. The plan contains training in bathing and the goal reads "patient will bathe with modified independence." It looks like there will not be any change in Mrs. Kelly's abilities so interventions are not warranted. The words utilized in therapy documentation must be read as they are and periodically examined objectively to ensure communication is effective and accurate.

Independence is not a one-time event because, by definition, the patient would be able to perform the task whenever he or she needed to. As an example, the patient may be able to stand up from his favorite recliner chair without incident in the morning when he is well rested but by afternoon he struggles and needs assistance when fatigue sets in. He is not truly independent with that specific transfer as he cannot complete it consistently. Therapists will be asked to see patients at times of the day when performance tends to be better and avoid times when mobility is more challenging, but an accurate picture of patient performance and developing a plan of necessary interventions is enhanced when the full scope of the difficulties the patient is having is observed.

Subjective information

Much like PLOF, the inclusion of subjective information is an integral part of a thorough therapy assessment. In conducting numerous record reviews, it appears that the amount of subjective information being collected is declining and in some cases completely absent.

As healthcare reform continues to reinforce the concept of patient-focused care, therapists need to pay attention to what patients have to say about their prior and current level of ability, how they feel about their situation, and what they hope to achieve by participating in therapy. Patients can, on occasion, talk for quite a long time about topics such as their bowels and it can be a challenge to help some of them focus on a particular question, but their participation in a therapy assessment is more than physical demonstration. Compliance with the ultimate plan of care is enhanced when the patient is part of the process and the goals of the individual are recognized and included.

Comprehensive Assessments

Completing assessments in the home setting carries with it the responsibility of managing an entire patient and not just one aspect of him or her. For therapists, this has raised concerns at times about what areas are in the scope of practice and what should be included in the documentation beyond the traditional elements of strength, mobility, and self-management. Before taking on those "therapy" areas in more detail, there are basic pieces of patient information that should be considered as part of routine assessments by any of the therapies practicing in home health.

Medical history

Recording the medical history of the patient creates the overall health status of the individual as well as outlines factors that may impact the course of care. Inclusion of the diagnosis codes being used for the home health episode show consistency of information with the overall plan of care.

Vital signs

Vital signs would include blood pressure, pulse, and respirations. Consideration should be given to temperature readings in patients identified with or prone to infections. Patient-specific parameters and criteria for physician notification should be communicated to all clinicians involved with the plan of care and be documented. These pieces of information provide insight into the general health of the patient and can be indicators of emerging issues of concern. Given the amount of activity that can occur during a therapy evaluation, readings pre- and postactivity as well as position change can provide important details as to the patient's status and reaction to treatment. Therapists need to be trained in how to take vital signs correctly and consistently, demonstrate competence, and be provided the appropriate equipment to complete these tasks.

Pain

Sometimes referred to as the fifth vital sign, assessment of pain extends beyond collecting data using the zero to 10 pain scale. Many patients are so accustomed to being asked to provide a number in a variety of healthcare settings that they will volunteer "I am a five" without even having to be asked. The current level of pain, what impacts it, and what patients are doing to manage it are areas present on nearly every therapy evaluation form, but at times this is left blank. Connecting back to Outcome and Assessment Information Set (OASIS), the additional component is the determination of how pain is impacting the ability of the patient to function. Has any activity or task been done less often or stopped completely in an attempt to manage pain? This can have specific relevance to physical therapy, occupational therapy, and speech-language pathology and increases the connectivity of traditional therapy assessments to meaningful patient information.

Medications

The therapist should look over the medication profile to determine if there are any potential issues that could impact the therapy plan of care. With some medications, side effects include fatigue and weakness and neither may be corrected with only a routine exercise program. A discussion of medication review is in the OASIS chapter of this book. At a fundamental level, it is important to consider the functionality of properly taking medications—ambulation skills to access them, fine motor skills to handle them, and cognitive skills to remember when and how to take them. Any changes in the regimen with respect to dose, frequency, or addition/removal of a medication should be documented according to agency policy.

Wounds

Inclusion of information about the presence of a wound or wounds is not directly implying that active wound care is part of the therapy plan. If there is a wound, the location and status could directly impact the ability of the patient to tolerate therapy activities. Precautions such as not getting the area wet could impact self-care issues. Specific to pressure ulcers, their existence may indicate a need to improve mobility to promote healing. If a risk for pressure ulcers has been assessed, minimizing or eliminating the contributing factors increases the support for addressing these issues through skilled therapy services.

Incontinence

The presence of incontinence may indicate physiological issues, but the underlying cause may be more related to mobility and self-care. The patient who is new to the use of a walker may find gait velocity decreased or that the walker does not fit easily through the doorways in the home. These delays can be the trigger for bladder "accidents" that were not an issue in the past. New onset of fatigue or weakness can contribute to challenges with toileting hygiene as well as fall risk when performing these tasks. Cognitive and communication issues can disrupt a timed voiding program or make it more difficult to know when the patient needs to be taken to the bathroom. These are very real and functional issues for patients, and each therapy can bring a set of skills to the table depending on the findings of the assessment.

Inclusion of these assessment areas, among others, may feel like an attempt to move "nursing" issues over to the therapies. The phrase "I just want to be a therapist" needs to be thought through carefully. A person is not "just a knee" or "just a stroke," and effective management of each individual begins with an assessment that looks at a broad range of issues and screens for potential problems that would warrant collaboration with other disciplines.

Connecting the Dots

A traditional therapy assessment covers all the basic areas of measurement—such as strength, balance, range of motion, and cognition, to name a few—by providing a separate and distinct area for each. In other areas of the form, whether electronic or on paper, sections for functional activities such as ambulation, dressing, bathing, swallowing, and memory will be found depending on the specific discipline completing it. There is an inherent assumption that the reader of the assessment will know which deficits connect to each functional problem. The question is, how well does that actually work in terms of communicating the unique skill set of each therapy discipline? The therapist needs to consider the need to be a more thorough job in connecting the dots (Figure 5.1).

FIGURE 5.1	Connecting the dots

Measurements	Functional impact
• Range of motion	• Ambulation
• Strength	• Transfers
• Balance	• Bathing
• Vision	• Dressing
• Pain	• Toileting
• Sensation	• Incontinence
• Communication	• Medication management
• Cognition	• Swallowing
• Environment	• Home management
• Equipment	

Consider these examples:

+ Patient A requires moderate assistance to shower safely. He has macular degeneration that makes it difficult to clearly see the temperature controls. He also has a balance issue that causes him to rely heavily on steadying himself on the shower wall.

+ Patient B requires moderate assistance to shower safely. He fell in the shower a week ago and is very anxious about being in that situation again. He is in need of a transfer bench.

+ Patient C requires moderate assistance to shower safely. He had rotator cuff surgery recently and is unable to actively use his left arm at this time. He has significant pain issues and complains of some dizziness after taking his medications.

In all three situations, the patient requires moderate assistance to shower safely but the reasons for this level of assistance vary greatly, just as would the plans to address them. The issue is that many current therapy evaluations stop at the level of designating the assistance and do not connect it to the measurable components that are causing the problems with a functional task. This contributes to assessments that contain limited skilled detail and can appear repetitive in nature upon review. It is the skills and experience of the therapist that see beyond the single piece of information that is the level of assistance that nontherapists may not see. These details are what makes the assessment distinctly therapy and show the indispensability of the care that is specific to each individual patient. Consideration of new tool formats or adaptations of current ones can be a key element in improving the content of therapy assessments and supporting medical necessity.

Tests and Measures

One clear message of the Home Health Prospective Payment System (PPS) 2011 Final Rule is the expectation for therapists to utilize tests and measures and document findings using these tools. In any discussion of this topic, understanding some key terminology is required. "Standardized" indicates that there is a defined way in which the assessment is completed and that it is followed every time the data is collected. Examples would be manual muscle testing and range of motion assessments. "Validated" tools have research behind them to support that the scoring or findings mean something real and are not random data. It is important to look into the available research to determine the patient population, like community-dwelling elderly, to confirm relevance to the patient the tool is being utilized with. Clarity around "standardized" and "validated" has been a challenge in home health specifically in relation to fall risk assessments. When OASIS-C became mandatory in 2010, item M1910 began to collect data about the use of fall risk assessment tools. In order to respond "yes" to this item, the tool had to be confirmed to be standardized (nearly all of the tools were) and validated for community-dwelling elderly (no single tool was by itself). Agencies expressed frustration having to respond "no" to M1910 because the tool they used for years was not validated according to these criteria.

Keep in mind that the reference to tests and measures for therapy in PPS 2011 do not require that they are both standardized and validated or that they are specific purchased tools. The criteria of OASIS M1910 do not directly apply here. Selection of tools is at the discretion of the therapist completing the assessment, and care should be taken to select ones that provide meaningful information and are actively used in care planning and not simply completed to meet a requirement. In addition, the completion of a test or measurement at the time of the initial assessment would warrant a repeat of the process at a point later on in the episode, minimally at the time of discharge, to confirm the impact of care. A measurement taken that is not repeated misses an opportunity to show patient progress.

Therapy-Specific Assessments

Moving into the therapy-specific assessment areas will impact each of the three therapies differently. Although one discipline may focus on an area more than another, it is imperative that there is a degree of consistency in the message being created about the patient when more than one therapy is providing care. Inconsistency creates the seeds of doubt about the accuracy of the assessment and can lead to denials of payment. As an example, the occupational therapist documents that the patient is ambulating "ad lib" in the home with no equipment or safety concerns. Meanwhile, the physical therapist is documenting a plan for eight visits to address fall risk and the need for gait training with a cane. As the payer source, one would lean toward the assessment of the occupational therapist and deny the need for physical therapy. This is not to say that clearly identical information would be present in all three therapy assessments, but support for the inclusion of the other services is a fundamental component of supporting the need for skilled intervention as a team.

The following are several key areas specific to physical therapy, occupational therapy, and speech-language pathology assessments. This is not an all-inclusive list as there can and should be variation in specific patient populations, but it is meant to facilitate improved transition from clinical decision-making to documentation to support medical necessity.

Physical therapy

Gait

Skilled gait assessments include the elements of the quality of the performance and not just the distance and device used. Assessment of stride length, weight shift, cadence, pelvic tilt, and balance are all examples of quality-related topics. Distance alone does not indicate there is a deficit that must be addressed. As an example, although 30 feet appears to be limited, the reason behind the limitation and why physical therapy is needed to correct this issue is not supported. It does not automatically require the skills of physical therapy to have a patient walk a longer distance because a caregiver could do that. Thirty feet could be an adequate distance in a one-room dwelling, but may not be adequate if the patient resides in an assisted living environment. It appears to be a practice for some of the physical therapists to omit distances completely from gait assessments. When distance is removed, there is no measurable frame of reference and limited functional context for ambulation. A skilled gait assessment is a balance of both the quality and the quantity of ambulation.

Transfers

There are a variety of possible transfers within this assessment area because it is more than the act of moving from a sitting to a standing position. The specific type of transfer, any relevant environment components, level of assistance required, contributing factors, and the steps involved combine to reflect the skills of the therapist. An outline of the key aspects of each transfer follows, but it is not an exhaustive list. Assessment would contain those relevant to the patient situation.

- Sit to stand transfer (recliner or kitchen chair)

  - Surface height

  - Use of support surfaces such as armrests

  - Position of feet

  - Ability to scoot forward

  - Ability to weight shift

  - Need for assistance (including "why")

  - Number of attempts

  - Fluidity of movement

  - Ability to return to sitting position

  - Safety throughout the task

- Tub/shower transfer

  - Ability to position self for the transfer

  - Use for/need for equipment

  - If done from seated position, include components of sit to stand transfer

  - Need for assistance (including "why")

  - Fluidity of movement

  - Ability to exit the tub/shower

  - Safety throughout the task

- Toilet transfer

  - Surface height

  - Use of support surfaces such as grab bars or counters

  - Position of self in front of toilet

  - Ability to sit down smoothly and safely

  - Need for assistance (including "why")

  - Number of attempts

  - Fluidity of movement

  - Ability to return to standing position

  - Safety throughout the task

- Bed to chair transfer

  - Ability to move from supine to a sitting position inclusive of level of assist and why assist is needed

  - Ability to stabilize self in seated position at edge of bed

  - Ability to shift weight properly

  - Use for/need for equipment

  - Need for assistance (including "why")

  - Ability to position self in front of next seating surface

  - Ability to return to sitting inclusive of level of assist and why assist is needed

  - Safety throughout the task

- Other transfers to consider

  - Car transfers: key to ability to access medical care outside the home

  - Getting up from the floor: important aspect of fall recovery training

  - Wheelchair transfers: use of a wheelchair as part of transfers will change some of the components and should be documented with that level of detail

Bed mobility

Assessment of bed mobility is often documented by level of assistance only. Ability to turn and position self in bed contains the components of rolling, bridging, and scooting. The "why" behind the level of assist may vary between components and should be documented when this is a problem area for a patient.

Fall risk

The risk for falls is based on multiple factors and is not confirmed by gait distances or a general scoring of balance as F-. Each patient has a unique set of risk factors, and these are what should drive the selection of interventions to decrease risks in a meaningful way. Factors include but are not limited to:

+ Medication regimen

+ Environmental issues

+ Weakness

+ Balance deficits

+ Visual issues

+ Cognitive issues

+ History and context of previous falls

+ Dizziness/vertigo

Self-care

Although some may assert that these areas are addressed more specifically by occupational therapy, the prevalence of this information being "deferred to occupational therapy" to that therapist or omitted completely misses an opportunity to connect deficit areas with functional issues. In addition, inclusion of this area supports the need for a referral to occupational therapy with objective data. Attention must be paid to why assistance is needed in the areas such as dressing, bathing, meal preparation, and medication management.

Balance

Formal test are used more often in this area of the physical therapy assessment and include but are not limited to the Tinetti, the Berg Balance Assessment, the Timed up and Go, and the 6-Minute Walk Test. These serve a much clearer purpose than general comments of "good," "fair," and "poor." Physical therapists must follow the standardization of these tools and cannot modify them on their own. It is important to confirm competence and comfort level with any tool selected, keeping in mind that a variety can be used.

Strength

Current documentation of manual muscle testing at times appears to be more of a screening than a true muscle-by-muscle formal assessment. This does not make a screening inappropriate but the therapist should be clear that testing muscle groups is not the same as isolated testing. The screening model should be a trigger for a more detailed assessment as indicated. "Muscle weakness" is not an observation but must have measurable data behind it as well as a clear connection to the impact on a meaningful functional activity.

Muscle tone

Although deemed to not be an issue for many home health patients, it may actually be overlooked. Inactivity can lead to atrophy over time and, in the increasing population of patients who are of very advanced age entering home health, one wonders if this component of a physical therapy assessment is being utilized correctly.

Range of motion

Documentation of both active and passive range of motion requires goniometry utilizing specified landmarks for any joint being assessed. This method meets the expectation of a standardized assessment. Estimating, eye-balling, or labeling "within functional limit (WFL)" does not. Tools that indicate measurements to the level of the toe joints were actually regularly taken by the physical therapist as part of the assessment raise questions as to relevance and accuracy. Focus should be on problem areas as indicated and how they impact function.

Endurance

Endurance has been turned into a dirty word in therapy circles based on the belief that use of it will trigger a payment denial. The issue is not the term itself but in how it has far too often been used in documentation. A classic example is an initial assessment that reads "Endurance: Fair" and a goal set for "Endurance will be good." Moving from fair to good sounds like a measurable improvement but key details are missing with respect to what the limited endurance is keeping the patient from doing and what additional endurance will mean for the patient's quality of life.

As opposed to addressing the core issues, a shift has been seen and encouraged by many to simply avoid the word endurance and replace it with "activity tolerance." The situation has not improved in any real way when records now read as assessments "Activity Tolerance: Fair" with a goal of "Activity tolerance will be good." The issue is this area has been a lack of clear connection to meaningful information from the patient's perspective. OASIS item M1400 reflects this issue in the area of dyspnea; the item asks for the level of activity that is provoking shortness of breath not tied to any specific pulmonary diagnosis. Therapy assessments should look at the dyspnea component of activity as well.

Edema

Circumferential measurements with consistent landmarks and specific descriptors such as pitting combined with any impact on mobility create a skilled assessment of edema beyond a "mild" or "moderate" designation.

Cognitive/behavioral

Issues with memory, alertness, depression, anxiety, and wandering are all relevant to successful execution of a physical therapy plan of care. Far too often the information stops at the level of "alert and oriented" but may be missing the opportunity to fully describe the complexities of the home health patient. The diagnosis label is not an actual assessment and, although focused interventions may not be a part of the plan, more detail is needed. The patient with depression may be feeling overwhelmed. The physical therapist may not be able to push this patient aggressively with respect to exercises and may need to keep the visits shorter to increase patient buy in.

The end result would be shorter visits compared to other patients and may lead to more total visits in order to effectively manage this patient. Given the current environment in which the provision of more therapy visits is questioned as being driven by reimbursement, physical therapists must be clear in how cognitive and or behavioral issues are impacting the plan of care.

Communication/comprehension

The ability of a patient to hear and understand communication as well as to respond appropriately is a critical component to effective teaching strategies and is often overlooked in physical therapy assessment documentation. It appears that ownership of teaching as a key element of therapy interventions is not being documented consistently. Acknowledgement of any factors that could impede this aspect or will call for adjustments in delivery—such as less verbal and more written communication or the need to use pictures as opposed to words—increases the ability to demonstrate the set of skills necessary to manage the home health patient.

Environment

The home health physical therapist knows the impact of the patient's environment on the ability to function more clearly than in other settings. The ability to ambulate in unobstructed, well lit, linoleum-covered hallways in a facility does not automatically translate to the home where clutter, throw rugs, and pets can add a whole new dynamic. Oxygen tubing can create exciting challenges to maneuvering a walker especially when the beloved cat finds the dangling tube very interesting. These factors are very real issues for the patient and relevant information that is well documented supports the need for a skilled therapist to be involved with the plan of care.

Safety

A consistent message of OASIS has been the "safety" of the patient when performing functional tasks. The challenge is defining safety in a way that is patient-specific and meaningful. Simply calling something safe or unsafe is not sufficient. The factors that are making a task safe versus unsafe must be included to reflect the skills of the therapist. Think about it this way: what is "safe" ambulation? For one patient safety is maintained by using a walker and having two people assist. For another it is the proper use of a cane when walking outdoors. For a third proper footwear is a key element because walking in slippers makes him unsteady and at risk for falls. The prevalence of fall prevention programs and the referrals specific to physical therapy to address very real risk issues should be a launching point for the level of detail required. The term "safe" does not stand alone as a measurement.

Vision

Much like cognition and communication, visual issues can have a direct impact on both functional ability and teaching strategies. This is not limited to more obvious challenges such as blindness. Consider how macular degeneration in the diabetic patient or light sensitivity can impact gait outdoors. The home program materials may need to be modified in order to be effective. This may not be a specific physical therapy treatment area, but it adds to the description of the unique and complex issues facing home health patients.

Sensation

Evaluation of sensation was taught as a basic component of physical therapy assessments starting back in school. Review of records shows a current tendency toward "intact" or "impaired" as the dominant response with no additional information. Screening for issues is important because a patient may not recognize a loss of sensation that has been gradually increasing over time. In addition, less than normal proprioception can be a significant contributing factor to gait issues and fall risk. The prevalence of diabetes reported for the home health population raises questions of underreporting of neuropathy issues by physical therapy as it is unclear if assessment for such is routinely occurring. OASIS-C added the process measure related to management of diabetic feet, which highlights the interest of Medicare in how this issue is being dealt with in the home setting. Physical therapy should be an active participant in this area, and sensation assessments are a key element of being part of the interdisciplinary team.

Key Assessment Concepts and Examples

Physical Therapy

Gait: include more than distance, device, and level of assistance

- Patient ambulates 75 feet with walker and stand-by assist (SBA) on level surface requiring 50% verbal cues to increase stride length on the right. Decreased swing phase on right limited by pain and weakness in the quadriceps. Time to complete distance is four minutes, 20 seconds.

- Patient requires moderate assistance to negotiate five steps with handrail to enter/exit the home due to inability to recall proper sequencing and weight-bearing restriction on lower left extremity of toe touch weight bearing.

- Patient ambulates 80 feet with contact guard assist (CGA) on lawn attempting to access the unattached garage which is 120 feet from the back door of the home. Increased unsteadiness noted on softer surfaces requiring a verbal cue 25% of the time for proper foot placement.

Transfers: consider the components of each specific transfer

- Sit to stand: Patient requires 50% verbal cues to scoot forward and position feet correctly and minimal assist with weight shift and coming to stand. Distractions in the environment such as the television or conversation increase need for verbal cues to 75% and two to three attempts to complete task correctly.

- Tub/shower transfer: Patient currently does not have a transfer bench and requires maximum assistance to enter and exit the shower area due to weakness in bilateral lower extremities (LE). Patient very anxious during the transfer due to fall in the shower two weeks ago.

- Toilet transfer: Patient is independent with a commode frame positioned over the toilet in the bathroom. No obstacles noted, and technique is appropriate without safety concerns.

Bed mobility: outline challenges to specific aspects

- Rolling: Patient is able to roll to right and left with 75% verbal cues for positioning of LEs and reaching properly for the railings.

- Scooting: Patient requires moderate assistance to scoot up in bed due to softness of the mattress and the lack of bed railings. A hospital bed is recommended.

Fall risk: connect specific risks to need for physical therapy

- Tinetti score is 16. Issues are more with respect to gait than balance, especially when changing directions.

- Patient at risk for orthostatic hypotension due to current medications. Needs verbal cues with all position changes to pause and wait before moving. When verbal cues not provided, movements are often quick and approximately 25% of the time result in complaining of symptoms of dizziness.

Self-care: ability to ambulate and transfer should connect to functional tasks

- Patient requires SBA to maintain a steady standing position and can tolerate this for no more than 45 seconds. This issue impacts the ability to groom, which now has to be seated level.

- Patient requires both hands on the walker at all times when ambulating, which impacts her ability to gather items and prepare meals as balance issues increase if even one hand is free.

Balance: consider tests and movement beyond "poor, fair, good"

- Single leg stance: two seconds on right, unable on left

- Timed up and go: 30 seconds

- Functional reach: unable with assistance

Strength: use actual measurements and connect to function

- Right quadriceps 3/5 decreasing swing phase of gait

- Left dorsiflexors 2/5 contributing to inability to clear left foot during gait

- Hip extensors 3/5 bilaterally and patient requires moderate assist to stand

Muscle tone: consider the impact of immobility

- Moderate decrease in tone of bilateral triceps noted. Minimum assistance needed with sit to stand transfer.

- Minimal hypertonicity in left calf during gait decreasing heel strike.

Range of motion: goniometry of specific joints connected to functional issues

- Right knee flexion 45 degrees limiting ability to position foot correctly for transfers

- Left knee extension lacks 20 degrees and seen in swing phase issues during gait

Endurance: utilize dyspnea as indicated and connect to functional task

- Dyspnea limits tolerance for gait to 45 feet. Patient is able to recover with standing rest break of one minute.

- Patient requires minimal assistance to ascend seven total stairs with onset of moderate dyspnea after three stairs completed.

Edema: include circumferential measurements, descriptors, and functional impact

- Right knee edema noted as circumferential measurement is 4 cm greater than the left and is limiting full active range of motion (AROM)

Cognitive/behavioral: consider impact on plan of care

- Patient's ability to comply with total hip precautions is limited by moderate dementia that requires 75% to 80% verbal cues during gait.

- Patient reports feeling overwhelmed with the amount of people coming to her home providing care. Discussed starting physical therapy at twice a week and reassess tolerance in two weeks.

Communication/comprehension: consider impact on education

- Home program materials need to be in picture format to improve quality of follow-through

- Moderate receptive aphasia requires the caregiver be an active participant in all physical therapy sessions to ensure consistent follow-through

Environment: focus on what is unique to the patient situation

- The position of the bed along the wall interferes with the safety and effectiveness of the transfer. Discussed the need to reposition with the patient and her daughter and they are in agreement.

- Ambulation to/from the bathroom is impacted by shag carpeting that makes use of the front wheel walker (FWW) more difficult for the patient.

Safety: determine what makes the task or activity "safe" or "unsafe"

- Patient requires moderate assistance of two to complete a safe sit to stand transfer

- Safety awareness ambulating around obstacles in the home is poor with one loss of balance stepping over a toy requiring moderate assistance to stabilize and two instances of bumping the walker into doorways

Vision: consider impact on function and plan of care

- Poor lighting in the living area makes navigation with FWW more problematic due to macular degeneration.

- Patient is unable to clearly read the discharge instructions from the hospital due to small size of print. Recommend use of spouse's magnifying glass, which helps significantly.

Sensation: screen for problems that impact function as well as other issues

- Proprioception is limited in left hip and knee, impacting patient's ability to place left leg properly when ambulating.

- Decreased sensation to light touch present in bilateral feet. Will incorporate teaching patient to monitor status of feet postambulation due to diagnosis of diabetes.

Occupational therapy

Activities of daily living (ADL)

It is vitally important that occupational therapists speak to individual self-care tasks and do not make generalized statements such as "min assist with ADLs." This practice misses the opportunity to clearly demonstrate the potential variability in performance of tasks relevant to specific patients. In all of these activities, a complete assessment requires more than the level of assistance and must include "why" there is an issue. ADLs include but are not limited to:

- **Grooming:** Attention to cognitive and mobility components that can impact ability to safely groom.

- **Dressing:** As with OASIS, consider the ability to gather the clothing items. Be aware of clothing choices to determine if the items are what the patient routinely wears or are a modification based on difficulties encountered.

- **Bathing:** There are several components within this task, so highlight the ones that are an issue such as reaching a specific region of the body. Do not overlook any complicating factors such as equipment needs, environmental concerns, or patient anxiety about bathing.

- **Toileting hygiene:** OASIS-C added a specific question in relation to ability to manage this important area of self-care, yet many occupational therapy documentation tools do not contain a distinct area for this information. Fall risk can be increased when there are limited abilities in this set of tasks and the connection to this increases the need for therapy interventions.

- **Medication management:** As mentioned in the OASIS chapter, medication management is not exclusively about knowledge of side effects and timing of doses. Cognitive issues that impact these areas can and should be addressed by occupational therapy. When assessing fine motor skills, the routine inclusion of specifics in relation to opening medication bottles or handling syringes would enhance the overall functional relevance of therapy interventions.

- **Feeding:** Assessment of self-feeding skills is not limited to neurologically impaired patients. Weakness or sensory issues in the upper extremities or sitting balance deficits can impact this area significantly.

Instrumental activities of daily living (IADL)

As with ADLs, specificity and relevance are key components to a thorough occupational therapy assessment. In all of these activities, a complete assessment requires more than the level of assistance and must include "why" there is an issue. IADLs include but are not limited to:

+ **Meal preparation:** There are many components to this task and with that comes multiple opportunities for issues to arise. Occupational therapists have known for a long time that food does not shoot out of refrigerator doors completely ready. Gathering, carrying, preparing, and transporting of food items can directly connect to fall risk and should be addressed as specific components.

+ **Money management:** This area can be related to a patient's sense of self-worth and is clearly meaningful in some cases. Assessment can reflect cognitive and communication issues as well.

+ **Household management:** Laundry, cleaning house, and managing home repair needs appear to often be dependent activities for home health patients based on the content of documentation. Clarity as to assessment as patient or caregiver report versus actual demonstration is important. Without detail, the impression is given that all of these tasks were attempted over the course of a single visit which would be unrealistic in nearly all cases.

Functional mobility

There has been a periodic debate between physical and occupational therapists about the inclusion of gait-related information in an occupational therapy assessment. Although physical therapy takes the lead on a detailed gait assessment, patients do walk during the course of many ADLs and IADLs and lack of any mobility information can make an occupational therapy assessment look incomplete.

Caution should be taken to avoid generalized statements that may negatively impact the medical necessity of physical therapy such as "patient ambulates ad lib," "patient ambulates independently," or "patient is independent with his cane" unless these are completely accurate based on the definition of independent previously discussed. Challenges and concerns with mobility noted during ADLs should be noted and coordinated with other disciplines.

Transfers

There are a variety of possible transfers within this assessment area because it is more than the act of moving from a sitting to a standing position. The specific type of transfer, any relevant environment components, level of assistance required, contributing factors, and the steps involved combine to reflect the skills of the therapist. An outline of the key aspects of each transfer follows, but it is not an exhaustive list. Assessment would contain the ones relevant to the patient situation.

- Sit to stand transfer (recliner or kitchen chair)

  - Surface height

  - Use of support surfaces such as armrests

  - Position of feet

  - Ability to scoot forward

  - Ability to weight shift

  - Need for assistance (including "why")

  - Number of attempts

  - Fluidity of movement

  - Ability to return to sitting position

  - Safety throughout the task

- Tub/shower transfer

  - Ability to position self for the transfer

  - Use for/need for equipment

  - If done from seated position, include components of sit to stand transfer

  - Need for assistance (including "why")

- Fluidity of movement

- Ability to exit the tub/shower

- Safety throughout the task

• Toilet transfer

- Surface height

- Use of support surfaces such as grab bars or counters

- Position of self in front of toilet

- Ability to sit down smoothly and safely

- Need for assistance (including "why")

- Number of attempts

- Fluidity of movement

- Ability to return to standing position

- Safety throughout the task

• Bed to chair transfer

- Ability to move from supine to a sitting position inclusive of level of assist and why assist is needed

- Ability to stabilize self in seated position at edge of bed

- Ability to shift weight properly

- Use for/need for equipment

- Need for assistance (including "why")

– Ability to position self in front of next seating surface

– Ability to return to sitting inclusive of level of assist and why assist is needed

– Safety throughout the task

+ Other transfers to consider

– Car transfers: key to ability to access medical care outside the home

– Getting up from the floor: important aspect of fall recovery training

– Wheelchair transfers: use of a wheelchair as part of transfers will change some of the components and should be documented with that level of detail

Bed mobility

Assessment of bed mobility is often documented by level of assistance only. Ability to turn and position self in bed contains the components of rolling, bridging, and scooting. The "why" behind the level of assist may vary between components and should be documented when this is a problem area for a patient.

Fall risk

The risk for falls is based on multiple factors and is not confirmed by gait distances or a general scoring of balance as F-. Each patient has a unique set of risk factors, and these are what should drive the selection of interventions to decrease risks in a meaningful way. Factors include but are not limited to:

+ Medication regimen

+ Environmental issues

+ Weakness

+ Balance deficits

+ Visual issues

    • Cognitive issues

    • History and context of previous falls

    • Dizziness/vertigo

Balance

Issues with balance in sitting and standing can have a significant impact on a variety of self-care tasks. Care should be taken with "poor," "fair," and "good" in relation to meaningful activity. For example, how would a patient with "poor" sitting balance be able to toilet independently? The larger picture of function must be kept in mind when this information is collected.

Strength

Occupational therapists have a similar risk when documenting strength to physical therapy. Current documentation of manual muscle testing at times appears to be more of a screening than a true muscle-by-muscle formal assessment. This does not make a screening inappropriate, but the therapist should be clear that testing muscle groups is not the same as isolated testing. The screening model should be a trigger for a more detailed assessment as indicated. "Muscle weakness" is not an observation but must have measurable data behind it as well as a clear connection to the impact on a meaningful self-care or household management activity.

Muscle tone

Although deemed to not be an issue for many home health patients, it may actually be overlooked. Inactivity can lead to atrophy over time and, in the increasing population of patients who are of very advanced age entering home health, one wonders if this component of an occupational therapy assessment is being utilized correctly.

Range of motion

Documentation of both active and passive range of motion requires goniometry utilizing specified landmarks for any joint being assessed. This method meets the expectation of a standardized assessment. Estimating, eye-balling, or labeling "WFL" does not. Tools that indicate measurements to the level of each individual finger joint were actually regularly taken by the occupational therapist as part of the assessment raise questions as to relevance and accuracy. Focus should be on problem areas as indicated and how they impact specific functional tasks.

Endurance

Endurance has been turned into a dirty word in therapy circles based on the belief that use of it will trigger a payment denial. The issue is not the term itself but in how it has far too often been used in documentation. A classic example is an initial assessment that reads "Endurance: Fair" and a goal set for "Endurance will be good." Moving from fair to good sounds like a measurable improvement but key details are missing with respect to what the limited endurance is keeping the patient from doing and what additional endurance will mean for the patient's quality of life. As opposed to addressing the core issues, a shift has been seen and encouraged by many to simply avoid the word endurance and replace it with "activity tolerance." The situation has not improved in any real way when records now read as assessments "Activity Tolerance: Fair" with a goal of "Activity tolerance will be good." The issue is this area has been a lack of clear connection to meaningful information from the patient's perspective. OASIS item M1400 reflects this issue in the area of dyspnea because the item asks for the level of activity that is provoking shortness of breath that is not tied to any specific pulmonary diagnosis. Therapy assessments should look at the dyspnea component of activity as well.

Edema

Circumferential measurements with consistent landmarks and specific descriptors such as pitting combined with any impact on mobility create a skilled assessment of edema beyond a "mild" or "moderate" designation.

Cognition/communication/comprehension/psychosocial issues

Occupational therapists have a unique set of skills to not only assess these areas but to directly tie any concerns to meaningful functional activities. Issues relevant to the occupational therapist's assessment include but are not limited to:

- Alertness

- Orientation

+ Short-term memory

+ Long-term memory

+ Ability to follow one-step commands

+ Ability to follow multiple-step commands

+ Judgment

+ Attention

+ Receptive language skills

+ Expressive language skills

+ Depression

+ Anxiety

Environment

The home health occupational therapist knows the impact of the patient's environment on the ability to function more clearly than in other settings. The ability to access a bathroom that clearly used to be a closet or kitchen appliances that are rather old and of questionable safety can add excitement to self-care training. Caring for a beloved pet is an IADL that the patient may care about more than any of the activities he or she practiced in the facility prior to discharge. Family dynamics can add a whole new dimension to managing dressing and meal preparation as roles in the home may be temporarily or permanently altered based on recent events. These factors are very real issues for the patient and relevant information that is well documented supports the need for a skilled therapist to be involved with the plan of care.

Safety

A consistent message of OASIS has been the safety of the patient when performing functional tasks. The challenge is defining safety in a way that is patient-specific and meaningful. Simply calling something safe or unsafe is not sufficient. The factors that are making a task safe versus unsafe must be included to reflect the skills of the therapist. Think about it this way: what is "safe" household management? First and foremost, that statement does not contain any specific details as to the task. For one patient safety when doing laundry is maintained by having one person assist carrying the clothes to the washing machine. For another, the patient may use her walker to transport the clothing but needs assistance to place them in the washing machine. For a third, the patient may have trouble remembering all of the steps involved in the correct order. The term "safe" does not stand alone as a measurement.

Sensorimotor

Much like the cognitive and communication category, there are many relevant pieces on information contained in a thorough occupational therapy assessment that have direct bearing on meaningful functional tasks. Sensorimotor areas include but are not limited to:

- Vision

- Hearing

- Neglect

- Body scheme

- Motor planning

- Left/right discrimination

- Spatial relationships

- Discerning figure/ground

Key Assessment Concepts and Examples

Occupational Therapy

Activities of daily living (ADL): focus on "why" the specific level of assistance is needed. ADLs include but are not limited to:

- Grooming
  - Patient requires constant verbal cues to correctly sequence brushing her teeth due to cognitive issues
  - Patient is dependent with combing her hair due to restriction to keep right arm in sling
- Dressing
  - Patient requires moderate assistance with upper body dressing due to poor sitting balance
  - Patient requires minimal assistance to complete lower body dressing secondary to pain issues limiting this activity
- Bathing
  - Patient is unable to shower at this time due to the bathroom being upstairs; the patient is currently restricted from using stairs per physician's order
  - Patient requires moderate assistance to shower due to anxiety from recent fall
- Toileting hygiene
  - Patient requires supervision with clothing management related to toileting due to mild unsteadiness when standing
  - Perianal hygiene: CGA to stabilize patient when leaning forward during the task
- Medication management
  - Patient's daughter is handling all aspects of medication management due to cognitive issues and several mistakes made by the patient in the last two weeks
  - Patient is unable to open medication bottles due to severe arthritis in both hands
- Feeding
  - Son provides supervision while patient feeds herself as recommended by the speech-language pathologist
  - Caregiver provides verbal cues to patient 50% of the time to take small sips when drinking thin liquids to prevent aspiration

Instrumental activities of daily living (IADL): focus on "why" the specific level of assistance is needed. IADLs include but are not limited to:

- Meal preparation
  - Patient requires moderate assistance to transport a plate of food from the counter to the table as she incorporates use of her new walker

     The How-to Guide to Home Health Therapy Documentation

- Use of microwave: supervision in order to perform the task in correct sequence and select appropriate cooking times

- Money management

  - Patient is currently unable to manage her checkbook due to exacerbation of memory issues.

  - Patient's daughter reports the patient frequently "forgets" where she has put her purse and has missed paying several bills on time over the last month. When asked to locate her purse, she was unable.

- Household management

  - Laundry: unable due to newly imposed non–weight-bearing status for right LE and need to use crutches when walking

  - House cleaning: Patient is able to wipe her kitchen counter after making a sandwich independently without loss of balance or pain interfering

- Functional mobility: address mobility impact on ADLs and IADLs

  - Patient ambulates from living room to bathroom with walker and SBA

  - Patient is dependent when utilizing a wheelchair when leaving the home

- Transfers: consider the components of each specific transfer

  - Tub transfer: moderate assistance to lift legs in to and out of the tub

  - Toilet transfer: CGA when standing up from the toilet due to complaint of dizziness when changing position

- Bed mobility: outline challenges to specific aspects

  - Rolling: Patient is able to roll to right and left with 75% verbal cues for positioning of LEs and reaching properly for the railings.

  - Scooting: Patient requires moderate assistance to scoot up in bed due to softness of the mattress and the lack of bed railings. A hospital bed is recommended.

- Fall risk: connect specific risks to need for occupational therapy

  - Patient does not have a transfer bench for the shower. Currently using shower rod as a grab bar and requires moderate assistance to complete the task. Significant risk for falling during this activity based on findings.

  - During meal preparation, patient noted to leave walker parked by the counter, which increases her level of unsteadiness when completing task.

- Balance: consider tests and movement beyond "poor, fair, good" while connecting issues to function

  - Dynamic sitting balance is fair. Patient requires moderate assistance to manage her shoes.

  - Patient is unable to perform functional reach due to dizziness when sitting longer than one minute. She will require maximum assistance when dressing at the side of the bed.

- Strength: use actual measurements and connect to function

  - Right shoulder flexion is 2/5 resulting in patient needing assistance with self-care

  - Left elbow flexion is 3/5 and limits ability to lift objects necessary for grooming

- Muscle tone: consider the impact of immobility

  - Moderate decrease in tone of bilateral triceps noted. Minimum assistance needed with sit to stand transfer.

  - Minimal hypertonicity in left biceps during tasks involving reaching for objects decreasing accuracy and requiring two to three attempts to complete.

- Range of motion: goniometry of specific joints connected to functional issues

  - Right elbow extension lacks 45 degrees, increasing the difficulty of the tub transfer

  - Thumb flexion limited to neutral impacting grip strength and functional use of left hand

- Endurance: utilize dyspnea as indicated and connect to functional task

  - Patient becomes short of breath twice during upper body dressing requiring a rest break of 30 seconds before proceeding

  - Dyspnea noted half way during showering, requiring an increased level of assistance from minimal to moderate to complete

- Edema: include circumferential measurements, descriptors, and functional impact

  - 1+ pitting edema present in right hand limiting full AROM and ability to grip the walker properly

- Cognition/communication/comprehension/psychosocial issues: connect concerns to functional tasks

  - Patient is able to consistently follow one-step commands but cannot handle multiple step commands. Instruction in meal preparation with the microwave will require verbal cues for safety.

  - Patient requires supervision during bathing due to level of anxiety.

- Environment: focus on what is unique to the patient situation

  - Patient's daughter is unwilling to assist with bathing as she is highly uncomfortable

  - Unable to assess bathing ability this visit as bathroom is currently being remodeled

- Safety: determine what makes the task or activity "safe" or "unsafe"

  - Safety awareness is fair during toileting and verbal cues needed to avoid using the toilet paper roll to push up

  - Patient requires the presence of another person throughout showering to ensure safety

- Sensorimotor: connect issues to functional tasks

  - Hearing: Patient requires increased volume when communicating verbally.

  - Mild left side neglect noted during grooming. Verbal cues needed to fully complete the task.

Speech-language pathology

Utilization of speech-language pathology services in home health has been directly impacted by staffing availability. Many agencies have learned to live with limited access to important discipline. Those that are in a unique situation with adequate, or dare say more than adequate staffing, may find themselves under review because practice patterns would be different when compared to other home health providers. Overall, the volume of therapy visits is predominantly made up of physical therapy, followed by occupational therapy, with speech-language pathology making up a smaller percentage of the total. This has nothing to do with importance or skill level but does put this specific therapy at a lower risk for targeted audit and denials because there are fewer total cases to pick from.

Speech-language pathologist assessments should cover more than swallowing and terms such as "impaired" without additional detail lack clarity as to the true scope of the issue. Assessment areas include but are not limited to the following:

- Oral motor function

    - Strength, range of motion, sensation, and function

- Swallowing

    - Posture, positioning, consistencies, and diet

- Cognition

    - Attention, orientation, recall, and memory

- Speech/language

    - Articulation, comprehension, hearing, and expression

One of the messages of 2011 home health PPS is the need for therapy to document information that is both measurable and meaningful. Anyone who has read a speech-language pathology assessment can become overwhelmed by the amount of measurable detail. There are often percentages, multiple and varied tests, and even the number of trials of gagging a patient with a frozen lemon glycerin swab. Of the three therapy disciplines, speech-language pathology generally outdoes the other two with respect to measurable information. There is a risk that must be addressed and cannot be overlooked: the connection to activities that are meaningful to the patient. As an example, Mr. Phillips is currently able to recall a series of verbal items with 70% accuracy. That sounds like a problem because 70% is less than 100% but does that clarify what the 30% difference in performance means for his ability to manage his new medications or to communicate with his spouse? As opposed to how the assessment information was presented for physical and occupational therapy, the examples will be of specific tool details to support the medical necessity of speech-language pathology. It has been noted on review of records that the quality of the assessment is highly influenced by the content of the documentation tool provided for this discipline, and agencies would be wise to assess current and future tools to reduce the risk of denials by facilitating complete assessments.

SPEECH PATHOLOGY: ORAL MOTOR EVALUATION   ( ) N/A

Dentition: ( ) WNL   ( ) Edentulous   ( ) Dentures   ( ) Poor Dentition   ( ) _____

Structure	WFL	Sensation	Strength	Range of Motion	Function
Facial CN VII		Absent/Decreased L/R/B		Rest: Symmetrical/Asymmetrical Smile: Symmetrical/Asymmetrical L/R/B	Impacts affect
Lips CN VII		Absent/Decreased L/R/B	Decreased Reduction in Closure Drooling L/R/B	Reduced Protrusion Reduced Retraction Decreased Rounding	Decreased Coordination Impaired Motor Planning
Tongue CN XII		Absent/Decreased L/R/B	Decreased L/R/B	Decreased Lateralization Decreased Protrusion Decreased Elevation Decreased Retraction	Decreased Coordination Impaired Motor Planning Tongue Fasciculations

Respiratory Status: ( ) WFL   ( ) SOB   ( ) Increased Rate   ( ) Accessory Muscle Use
( ) Decreased Breath Support   ( ) Short Rushes of Speech   ( ) Excessive Secretions
( ) Ventilator Dependent   ( ) Tracheostomy: Cuff/Cuffless: Size: 4   6   8
Capped/Speaking Valve/Finger occlusion/Fenestration

Voice / Airway Protection:

Quality: ( ) WNL   ( ) Aphonic   ( ) Breathy   ( ) Hoarse   ( ) Strained   ( ) Harsh
( ) Wet/Gurgly   ( ) Hypernasal   ( ) Hyponasal   ( ) Nasal Emissions ( ) Intermittent Phonation

Intensity: ( ) WNL   ( ) Fatigues with Use   ( ) Variable

Pitch/Intonation: ( ) WNL   ( ) Excess/Equal Stress   ( ) Monotone   ( ) Limited Variation

Voluntary Cough: ( ) WNL   ( ) Weak   ( ) Unable to Perform

Reflexive Cough: ( ) WNL   ( ) Weak/Nonproductive

SPEECH PATHOLOGY: CLINICAL SWALLOWING EVALUATION ( ) N/A

Current Method of Nutrition: ( ) Oral ( ) Regular ( ) Mech. Soft-Chopped meat /Ground Meat ( ) Pureed
( ) NPO ( ) IV ( ) NG/Dubhoff ( ) G-Tube ( ) J Tube

Posture/ Positioning: ( ) WFL ( ) Restricted: _____
( ) Self-Fed ( ) Assisted Feeding

Consistencies Tested: ( ) Liquids: ( ) Teaspoon ( ) Straw ( ) Cup
( ) Solids: ( ) Puree ( ) Soft Chewable ( ) Hard/Chewy consistency

Observations	Findings	Consistency
Drooling	Poor sensation/poor labial closure	
Leakage of food from mouth	Poor labial closure	
Slow oral transit time	Poor sensation/poor tongue movement	
Residue in front of mouth	Poor tongue movement	
Residue in back of mouth	Poor sensation	
Pocketing in L/R Buccal cavity	Poor tongue lateralization/decreased buccal tension/ decreased sensation	
Adherence to hard palate	Poor tongue elevation	
Tongue pumping	Decrease tongue control/coordination Decreased swallow initiation	
Increased chewing time	Decreased mandibular strength/decreased attention/ limited dentition	
Holding of food/liquid	Poor sensation /awareness/decreased initiation	
Coughing before swallow	Decreased oral control/possible aspiration/delayed initiation	
Coughing after swallow	Possible pharyngeal residue due to decreased laryngeal elevation, weak tongue base and/or cricopharyngeal opening-relaxation/possible aspiration/penetration	
Multiple swallows	Possible pharyngeal residue due to decreased laryngeal elevation, weak tongue base and/or cricopharyngeal opening-relaxation	
Wet Voicing	Penetration/possible aspiration	
Change in respiration / breath sounds	Penetration/possible aspiration	
Absent swallow response	Poor awareness/decreased sensation/decreased initiation	
Delayed swallow response: _____ seconds	Poor awareness/decreased sensation/decreased initiation	
Absent / Limited laryngeal excursion	Decreased laryngeal elevation	
Complaints of localized pain and /or "sticking"	Possible decreased esophageal motility/reflux	
Regurgitation	Possible reflux/ r/o diverticulum	
Other:		

Cognitive-Communication: ( ) WFL for this evaluation   ( ) Impacts swallow safety   ( ) Further evaluation warranted

Functional Limitations Include: ( ) Risk of aspiration   ( ) Risk of decreased nutrition/hydration   ( ) None

Diet Recommendations:

Solids: _____

Liquids: _____

Other: _____

Recommendations

( ) Therapeutic exercises	( ) Positioning strategies	( ) Compensatory strategies
( ) Oral motor/tongue base	( ) Upright position	( ) Feed slowly
( ) Bolus manipulation	( ) Upright minimum 1 hour post m	( ) Small bites/sips
( ) Vocal fold adduction	( ) Chin tuck	( ) Multiple swallow per bite
( ) Thermal stimulation	( ) Turn head R/L	( ) Tongue pressure with bite
( ) Other: _____	( ) Head tilt R/L	( ) Alternate liquid/solid
	( ) Other: _____	( ) Liquid wash at meal end

Other Recommendations:

( ) Refer for videofluroscopic swallow study

( ) Dietitian consult

( ) SLP to upgrade diet consistency as tolerated

( ) Caregiver/Family to supervise

( ) Five to six small meals a day

( ) Effortful swallow

( ) Mendelsohn maneuver

( ) Supraglottic swallow

( ) Super supraglottic swallow

( ) Other: _____

_____

SPEECH PATHOLOGY: SPEECH-LANGUAGE EVALUATION   ( ) N/A

Articulation / Speech Production: ( ) Functional   ( ) Not Tested   ( ) Further Evaluation Warranted

Overall Speech Intelligibility:
    ( ) WNL   ( ) Mild 80%–90%   ( ) Moderate 50%–79%   ( ) Mod-Severe 30%–49%   ( ) Severe 0%–29%

( ) Dysarthria: ( ) No intelligible speech   ( ) Apraxia: ( ) Nonverbal

( ) Produce intelligible syllables   ( ) Produces counting, singing

( ) Produces intelligible words   ( ) Produces automatic responses

( ) Produces intelligible 2–3 word phrases ( ) Produces single words

( ) Produces intelligible 7–10 word phrases ( ) Produces 2–3 word phrases

( ) Produces intelligible conversation but fatigues ( ) Produces sentences

( ) Produces intelligible conversational speech ( ) Initiates conversational speech

Comments: _____

_____

Auditory Comprehension: ( ) Functional   ( ) Not Tested   ( ) Further Evaluation Warranted

        ( ) No usable comprehension skills
        ( ) Max cues for simple one-step commands and simple yes/no questions
        ( ) Follows one-step commands/simple questions with moderate cues
        ( ) Follows one-step commands/simple questions with minimal cues
        ( ) Comprehends simple directions and conversation with contextual cues
        ( ) Comprehends complex conversation and directions but may need extra time to understand
        ( ) Understands complex and abstract directions and conversation without cues

Comments: _____

Hearing Status: ( ) Functional   ( ) Hard of Hearing   ( ) Hearing Aid (right/left/bilateral)   ( ) Assistive Device

Expressive Language: ( ) Functional   ( ) Not Tested   ( ) Further Evaluation Warranted
        ( ) Non verbal/nonmeaningful productions
        ( ) Uses automatic speech with maximal cues
        ( ) Produces words and phrases with moderate cues
        ( ) Initiates simple sentences with moderate cues
        ( ) Initiates spoken language in simple conversation with minimal cues
        ( ) Engages in general conversation
        ( ) Engages in complex conversation

Repetition: Words: ( ) WNL ( ) Mild 80%–90% ( ) Moderate 50%–79% ( ) Mod-Severe 30%–49% ( ) Severe 0%–29%
            Sentences: ( ) WNL ( ) Mild 80%–90% ( ) Moderate 50%–79% ( ) Mod-Severe 30%–49% ( ) Severe 0%–29%

Naming/Word Finding:
    Objects / picture: ( ) WNL ( ) Mild 80%–90% ( ) Moderate 50%–79% ( ) Mod-Severe 30%–49% ( ) Severe 0%–29%
    Categorization: ( ) WNL ( ) Mild 80%–90% ( ) Moderate 50%–79% ( ) Mod-Severe 30%–49% ( ) Severe 0%–29%
Sentence Completion: ( ) WNL ( ) Mild 80%–90% ( ) Moderate 50%–79% ( ) Mod-Severe 30%–49% ( ) Severe 0%–29%

Comments: _____

Reading / Writing Pre morbid Status: ( ) Functional   ( ) Limited   ( ) Nonreader/writer
Visual Aides: ( ) Glasses   ( ) Contacts   ( ) _____
Reading / Visual Comprehension: ( ) Functional   ( ) Not Tested   ( ) Further Evaluation Warranted
        ( ) No usable visual comprehension
        ( ) Comprehends letters and common words with maximal cues
        ( ) Comprehends single letters and common words with moderate cues
        ( ) Comprehends words and phrases in daily routines; moderate cues for sentences
        ( ) Comprehends sentences without cues and complex sentences with minimal cues
        ( ) Comprehends functional material with limitations
        ( ) Comprehends complex reading material

Quality: ( ) WNL   ( ) Blurry   ( ) Blind   ( ) Diminished Visual Field: R/L
          ( ) Impaired Scanning/Tracking   ( ) Responds to visual threat

Comments: _____

Written Expression / Writing: ( ) Functional   ( ) Not Tested   ( ) Further Evaluation Warranted
    ( ) No usable skills
    ( ) Copies letters/words
    ( ) Writes single words with cues
    ( ) Writes phrases and sentences with cues
    ( ) Writes simple paragraphs with cues
    ( ) Writes paragraphs and complex material with cues
    ( ) No limitations

Comments: _____

Cognitive-Communication: ( ) Functional   ( ) Not Tested   ( ) Further Evaluation Warranted
Integrative Language:
  Attention: ( ) Nonfunctional
           ( ) Briefly attends with maximal stimulation
           ( ) Completes simple tasks with maximal cues without distractions
           ( ) Completes multistep tasks with minimal distractions
           ( ) Completes simple living tasks with distractions and complex tasks with increased cues
           ( ) Completes complex tasks with minimal cues, may need increased time for multiple tasks
           ( ) No limitations

Orientation-location:	( ) WNL	( ) Mild 80-90%	( ) Moderate 50-79%	( ) Mod-Severe 30-49%	( ) Severe 0–29%
Orientation-time/day:	( ) WNL	( ) Mild 80-90%	( ) Moderate 50-79%	( ) Mod-Severe 30-49%	( ) Severe 0–29%
Immediate Recall:	( ) WNL	( ) Mild 80-90%	( ) Moderate 50-79%	( ) Mod-Severe 30-49%	( ) Severe 0–29%
Delayed Recall:	( ) WNL	( ) Mild 80-90%	( ) Moderate 50-79%	( ) Mod-Severe 30-49%	( ) Severe 0–29%
Long Term Memory:	( ) WNL	( ) Mild 80-90%	( ) Moderate 50-79%	( ) Mod-Severe 30-49%	( ) Severe 0–29%
Problem Solving:	( ) WNL	( ) Mild 80-90%	( ) Moderate 50-79%	( ) Mod-Severe 30-49%	( ) Severe 0–29%
Abstract Reasoning:	( ) WNL	( ) Mild 80-90%	( ) Moderate 50-79%	( ) Mod-Severe 30-49%	( ) Severe 0-29%
Organization/Sequencing:	( ) WNL	( ) Mild 80-90%	( ) Moderate 50-79%	( ) Mod-Severe 30-49%	( ) Severe 0–29%
Initiation:	( ) WNL	( ) Mild 80-90%	( ) Moderate 50-79%	( ) Mod-Severe 30-49%	( ) Severe 0–29%
Awareness of Deficit:	( ) WNL	( ) Mild 80-90%	( ) Moderate 50-79%	( ) Mod-Severe 30-49%	( ) Severe 0– 29%
Time Concepts:	( ) WNL	( ) Mild 80-90%	( ) Moderate 50-79%	( ) Mod-Severe 30-49%	( ) Severe 0–29%
Numbers / Money:	( ) WNL	( ) Mild 80-90%	( ) Moderate 50-79%	( ) Mod-Severe 30-49%	( ) Severe 0–29%

Pragmatics: ( ) Flat affect   ( ) Emotional labile
Topic Exchange: ( ) Verbose/hyperverbal   ( ) Limited maintenance of topic   ( ) Limited initiation of requests

Safety Awareness: ( ) WNL   ( ) Mild   ( ) Moderate   ( ) Mod–Severe   ( ) Severe   ( ) Not Tested
                    Patient able to recall safety precautions or therapist recommendations: ( ) Yes ( ) No ( ) NA
                    Patient independently utilizes assistive device ( ) Yes ( ) No ( ) NA

Comments: _____

Closing Thoughts

Completion of a thorough therapy assessment requires a comprehensive focus with attention to key details. Consideration of all the possible areas to be addressed can feel overwhelming and raise issues noted in previous chapters with respect to a general dislike of documentation. Shortcuts in this area may initially appear to be more efficient and time-saving, but the repercussions can far outweigh any perceived benefits if ultimately the decision is made that the services are not medically necessary. All other components of documentation—the goals, the plan of care, and the interventions delivered on subsequent visits—are all driven by the content and focus of the assessment. Care must be taken to generate documentation that clearly reflects the unique set of skills possessed by physical therapy, occupational therapy, and speech-language pathology and support the need for these disciplines to be involved in the plan of care for patients now and in the future.

Goals: Measurable and Meaningful

Just as therapy assessments create the foundation for the plan of care, goal statements provide a vision of the ultimate structure and guide the process of putting the plan together. There is a common misconception that a set of therapy goals must include at least one specific statement related to strength, one for range of motion, and one for balance. There is no mandatory outline of goals that must be included for each therapy or a template that will work for all home health patients.

Therapy clarifications in Home Health Prospective Payment System 2011 indicate that goals should meet two primary criteria: measurable and meaningful. This is not new information to therapists in any setting and is not specific to Medicare regulations. Over time, content and direction of therapy goals risk becoming vague in terms of measurements combined with unclear functional relevance—both of which undermine the ability to support the medical necessity of therapy services. Keeping in mind the previous discussion of homebound status, goals must take into consideration the physical demands required to be mobile in the community. Setting high-level goals does negatively impact homebound status but creates the expectation of the level of function needed for the patient to return to his or her life. Once the goals are met, then the patient would no longer be considered homebound. Often, this is the driver behind the referrals to therapy services. Ownership of goal statements must be taken back by physical therapists, occupational therapists, and speech-language pathologists as a natural extension of a thorough assessment.

Measurable

Well-written goals correlate to assessment findings. The measurement component begins with consistent data collection and the incorporation of relevant standardized tests as indicated. The presence of a deficit in strength, range of motion (ROM), or cognition does not necessitate skilled therapy interventions or always translate into the potential to improve. Factors such as the length of time the patient has had the deficit and his or her willingness to work on improving the current situation are but two components of what is referred to as "rehabilitation potential" and must be taken into consideration when developing therapy goals. Goals must contain a measurement to reflect the impact of treatment on specific aspects of the skills and abilities of each unique patient.

Periodic rumors arise surrounding the use of measurements such as gait distances in physical therapy goals—the most common of which is that setting a target of greater than 150 feet will lead to a denial of payment. There is nothing currently in the regulations that resembles a list of any specific distances that put a record at risk. Envision a conference room at the Medicare office building in Maryland. The person leading the meeting is going over an agenda item about concerns of overutilization of physical therapy in home health. After some debate, the group decides that 149 feet of ambulation is acceptable and so is 150 feet, but if the distance goes to 151 feet or more an automatic denial will be given. Thinking logically, this scenario does not make sense. Issues regarding gait distance being perceived as too high have never been about the measurement in isolation but the reality that, for too many patients, gait-related goals rely on a higher distance than was possible at the assessment visit without a relevant functional context.

Measurements without meaning create incomplete goals such as these:

* Patient will ambulate safely 200 feet

    - "Safely" is not clearly defined with patient-specific details such as equipment use and/or level of assistance needed

    - Unable to determine what is important to the patient that requires 200 feet to access

* Patient will increase right shoulder ROM to within functional limits (WFL)

    - ROM is not defined in relevant terms of active or passive ROM

    - WFL does not connect ROM to a meaningful functional task that will be improved by this increase

- Increase speech intelligibility to 80%

  - Increase would indicate some improvement but the relevance of 80% is unclear

  - Intelligibility is not being connected to a specific meaningful task

Attention to useful and clear measurements must be maintained when creating goals, but they do not stand alone to support the medical necessity of therapy services.

Meaningful

Shifting gears to the component of meaningful in relation to goal statements requires a different starting point than measurable. Patients must be active participants in the creation of their plan of care and goals, and this is more than the statement "patient agrees with the plan of care." It is unlikely that a home health patient has actually stated the desire to "ambulate 200 feet with a walker and stand-by assistance." Appropriate goals contain information that is relevant and important to the patient and puts the therapy interventions into a meaningful context. It is possible to become too focused on the perception of functionality as seen in these examples.

- Patient will ambulate household distances with/without assistive device (AD) independently

  - Household is not defined and varies greatly depending on living situation. Without a standard definition there is no clear way to determine when the goal is reached.

  - With/without AD is problematic and should be one or the other with respect to use of an AD.

- Patient will complete home management skills safely

  - Home management is not task-specific, and it is unclear which components are going to be addressed

  - Safely is not a measurement and requires more patient-specific detail with respect to any equipment or level of assistance required

- Patient will demonstrate improved communication skills

    – Improved sounds meaningful but is not clearly defined by an actual measurement

    – Communication skills also sounds meaningful but is not specific in terms of components involved

With the increased attention on the need for therapy goals to be meaningful it is possible to unintentionally shift too far in that direction and omit measurable detail thus decreasing the ability to support medical necessity.

Finding Balance

Therapy goals require a balance between measurement and meaning. Both physical therapy and speech-language pathology goals have a tendency toward more solid measurements but may lack clear functional relevance. Supporting the functional relevance of goals should be patient-specific and not a standardized response such as linking all gait-related goals to accessing the mailbox. Occupational therapy goals have a strategic advantage with respect to being meaningful with tasks such as dressing, bathing, and meal preparation but can leave out measurements to show progress and support ultimate goal attainment.

Referring to activities of daily living (ADL) and instrumental ADLs (IADL) in groups as opposed to individual activities misses an opportunity to enhance the quality of the goals. Documentation tools that create standardized lists of goals from which the therapist can choose is intended to be a time-saving strategy but can lead to repetitive and less useful information. This is not to say the concept of a list is the problem, but there needs to be patient-specific customization of goal statements and critical thinking behind which ones are selected. Looking at a group of goals indicates that more is not always better, and there are times when goals are selected that are not supported by the assessment or are not reflected in the planned interventions. One size does not fit all for therapy goals, and the appropriate balance between measurable and meaningful requires and ultimately supports the skills of each specific therapy provided to the patient.

Goal examples

The examples provided are not meant to be used as cut and paste options for therapy records but are intended to provoke critical thinking about writing goal statements. Some aspects within a discipline may appear repetitive and in reality may actually be combined into a single goal statement but are separated as follows to highlight specific ideas. There is some overlap of areas between the therapies but this should not be automatically seen as duplication of services. The three therapies can and should work in partnership in several areas but the skills being utilized to address issues will be unique to each discipline and the documentation must reflect that level of detail.

Physical therapy

+ Gait: determine where the patient wants to go

    – Patient will ambulate 250 feet with walker independently on even and uneven surfaces to allow access to vehicle for transport from the home

    – Patient will ambulate 1000 feet with supervision to allow her to go grocery shopping with her granddaughter as was her prior level of function

+ Transfers: consider what improvement will allow the patient to do

    – Patient will complete sit to stand transfer independently pushing up from the armrests consistently to steady self

    – Patient will be able to get up from floor level with supervision as a fall recovery strategy

+ Bed mobility: include impact on caregivers

    – Patient will perform bridging with 25% verbal cues to assist caregiver with hygiene and dressing

    – Patient will roll bilaterally independently using bed railings as needed

- Fall risk: connect specific risks addressed by physical therapy

  - Patient will remove throw rugs from living areas to decrease risk of tripping when ambulating with walker

  - Patient's son will provide supervision when ambulating outdoors to decrease risk of falls based on periodic fatigue

- Self-care: ability to ambulate and transfer should connect to functional tasks

  - Patient will ambulate 50 feet independently to access her bathroom for toileting

  - Patient will be independent with wheelchair propulsion to 75 feet over carpet to access kitchen area for meals

- Balance: connect changes to function

  - Tinetti score will be 22 or higher indicating a minimal risk for falls

  - Single leg stance will be one minute to improve ability to ascend and descend steps in home to sleeping area

- Strength: use actual measurements and connect to function

  - Left lower extremity dorsiflexors will be 4/5 to improve toe clearance during swing phase of gait and decrease risk of tripping

  - Right knee extensors will be 4/5 to improve symmetrical step length during gait cycle

- Muscle tone: connect changes to functional tasks

  - Tone in left hamstrings will be normalized to increase knee active ROM (AROM) to WFL

  - Tone in right plantar flexors will be normalized to improve heel strike and decrease fall risk while ambulating

GOALS: MEASURABLE AND MEANINGFUL

- ROM: goniometry of specific joints connected to functional issues

  - Right knee flexion will be 100 degrees to allow for foot flat in seated position

  - Left knee extension will be to neutral to improve posture during standing and decrease c/o back pain

- Endurance: utilize dyspnea as indicated and connect to functional task

  - Patient will tolerate ambulation to 300 feet without symptoms of dyspnea to allow access to backyard to interact with her dog

  - Patient will ascend and descend five stairs independently without symptoms of dyspnea

- Edema: include functional impact

  - Edema will decrease in the left foot to allow for proper shoes to be worn when ambulating

  - Edema will decrease in the right knee to allow full AROM

- Cognitive/behavioral: consider impact on function

  - Patient will complete entire home program independently without anxiety being observed or reported.

  - Patient will verbally recall total hip precautions independently. Will require supervision to ensure compliance with same based on current level of memory issues.

- Communication/comprehension: consider impact on meaningful tasks

  - Patient will complete home exercise program with occasional verbal cues from her caregiver to ensure quality of performance

  - Patient will demonstrate use of communication board as directed by the speech-language pathologist to communicate needs during wheelchair mobility tasks

- Environment: focus on what is unique to the patient situation

- Patient's daughter will remove throw rugs from the bathroom to prevent tripping with the walker when accessing the toilet

- Patient will ambulate to 100 feet in the home independently with front wheel walker over moderately thick carpeting without loss of balance

• Safety: determine what makes the task or activity "safe" or "unsafe"

- Patient will ambulate 400 feet safely with supervision and a cane on uneven surfaces to allow access to bus stop in front of home

- Patient will transfer on and off the toilet independently with safe and consistent use of commode frame

• Vision: consider impact on function

- Patient will ambulate to 150 feet around home obstacles independently using her walker and compensating for blindness in left eye

- Patient will recall the need to turn on the lights in her home in the evenings to improve her ability to see potential trip hazards

• Sensation: connect to function

- Patient will be independent visually inspecting bilateral feet for pressure areas after ambulating for longer than 10 minutes due to decreased sensation as part of diabetic management

- Patient will independently recall the need to visually confirm foot placement on stairs due to issues with proprioception to decrease risk for falls

Occupational therapy

ADLs include but are not limited to:

• Grooming

- Patient will brush her hair independently while standing unsupported at the sink

GOALS: MEASURABLE AND MEANINGFUL

- Patient will complete teeth brushing with verbal cues for sequencing as indicated due to dementia

+ Dressing

- Patient will complete lower body dressing independently following total hip precaution with use of a dressing stick

- Patient will perform upper body dressing with intermittent moderate assistance for left arm only as she will be in a sling for the next two months

+ Bathing

- Patient will bathe independently with a shower chair in place

- Patient will bathe independently in a stand up shower utilizing a grab bar to steady self as needed

+ Toileting hygiene

- Patient will require supervision for clothing management during toileting due to right arm being immobilized

- Patient will complete perianal hygiene independently without loss of balance

+ Medication management

- Patient will demonstrate adequate fine motor skills to open medication bottles independently

- Patient will set up pill box independently and accurately

+ Feeding

- AROM of right arm will be WFL to allow patient to complete feeding independently

- Grip strength of left hand will be WFL to allow her to adequately hold a fork or spoon during self-feeding

IADLs include but are not limited to:

* Meal preparation

    - Patient will be able to reheat a plate of food in the microwave independently

    - Patient will independently transport a plate of food from the counter to the table while using her cane

* Money management

    - Patient will be able to locate her purse 80% of the time when asked by keeping it in one consistent location

    - Patient will require supervision during check writing to ensure accuracy

* Household management

    - Patient will be independent with laundry tasks, incorporating her walker correctly

    - Patient will wipe off the counter independently after meal preparation without loss of balance

* Functional mobility: address mobility impact on ADLs and IADLs

    - Patient will follow through with gait instructions from physical therapist during meal preparation activities.

    - Patient will require supervision when gathering her clothing items. Once collected, she will be independent with the task of dressing.

* Transfers: consider what improvement will mean to the patient

    - Patient will complete toilet transfer independently decreasing the workload of the caregiver

    - Patient will complete tub transfer independently using a transfer bench consistently

GOALS: MEASURABLE AND MEANINGFUL

+ Bed mobility: consider impact on caregivers

  – Patient will complete bridging independently to assist with lower body dressing

  – Patient will be able to change position in bed independently to decrease risk of pressure ulcers

+ Fall risk: connect specific risks to need for occupational therapy

  – Patient will demonstrate use of transfer bench during every bathing activity to decrease risk for falls

  – Patient will increase upper extremity strength to WFL to allow patient to push up from her chair instead of trying to pull up on walker to decrease risk for falls

+ Balance: consider tests and movement beyond "poor, fair, good" while connecting issues to function

  – Patient will be able to reach bilaterally to targets at varying distances in a seated position without loss of balance to improve ability to manage self-care from wheelchair level

  – Patient will stand independently unsupported for five minutes at the kitchen counter without loss of balance to allow participation in meal preparation

+ Strength: use actual measurements and connect to function

  – Increase strength of right elbow flexion to 5/5 to increase ability to feed self

  – Increase strength of bilateral elbow extension to 5/5 to decrease assist needed for sit to stand transfer to supervision

+ Muscle tone: consider the impact on functional ability

  – Flexor tone in right upper extremity will be normalized to decrease assistance needed for dressing and writing

  – Flexor tone in the left hand will decrease to allow initiation of appropriate splinting for contracture management

- Range of motion: goniometry of specific joints connected to functional issues

  - Right shoulder flexion AROM to 100 degrees to increase ability to groom

  - Left wrist extension AROM to neutral to gain proper hand position when using the walker

- Endurance: utilize dyspnea as indicated and connect to functional task

  - Patient will complete bathing task using tub seat with one rest break of less than two minutes to manage dyspnea

  - Patient will complete dressing activities incorporating pursed lip breathing skills without cues

- Edema: include circumferential measurements, descriptors, and functional impact

  - Edema in left hand will decrease to allow for full AROM and improve functional use of the hand

  - Patient will be independent in use of lower extremity compression stockings as part of edema management program

- Cognition/communication/comprehension/psychosocial issues: connect concerns to functional tasks

  - Patient will be able to independently prepare a meal requiring 10 to 15 steps without cues

  - Patient will demonstrate independent use of a diary to manage medications

- Environment: focus on what is unique to the patient situation

  - Patient will keep a set of dishes at counter level to remove need to reach into cabinets or use a step stool to access needed items

  - Patient will use a non-slip mat outside her shower whenever she is bathing to decrease fall risk upon exit

- Safety: determine what makes the task or activity "safe" or "unsafe"

- Patient will complete bathing independently and with good safety awareness as seen in use of transfer bench and handheld shower consistently

- Patient will require supervision during meal preparation due to safety concerns when handling cutlery

+ Sensorimotor: connect issues to functional tasks

- Patient will be independent using a modified phone due to her hearing impairment

- Patient will be independent reading medication labels with use of magnifying glass

Speech therapy

+ Oral motor function: strength, ROM, sensation, and function

- Patient will demonstrate normal lip closure at rest, and drooling will be absent

- Coordination of tongue movements will normalize during feeding to improve quality of the activity

+ Swallowing: posture, positioning, consistencies, and diet

- Patient will be independent with nectar consistency restrictions to decrease risk of aspiration

- Patient will utilize appropriate chin tuck during swallowing with supervision and occasional verbal cues

+ Cognition: attention, orientation, recall, and memory

- Patient will recall three- to five-step commands independently, which will improve her ability to recall information provided by her medical team

- Patient will demonstrate independent use of a calendar to keep track of appointments

• Speech/language: articulation, comprehension, hearing, and expression

  – Patient will demonstrate comprehension of complex written material such as the information provided with her prescriptions to promote safe medication management

  – Patient will be independent with communication board in making needs known and increased interaction with family members in social situations

Managing Goals

Any discussion of therapy goals raises questions about the model that should be used. There is a debate in home health about creating a single set of goals for the episode of therapy or establishing short- and long-term goals. From a regulatory perspective, there is nothing that specifies a required method to follow, which leaves the decision up to therapists. There are positives and risks associated with both options, as follows.

Long-term goals only

• Perception that it is easier to manage and ensure follow through with only one set of goals in place

• Decreased risk of missing a date adjustment as target is always the end of care

• Have a tendency to lack specific detail in order to cover a longer period of time

• Infrequent to see updates made over the course of care in response to patient progress or lack thereof

Short- and long-term goals

• Create intermediate targets by which to measure progress along the course of care

• Provide an opportunity to modify, as needed, when dates are met or extensions are needed

• Tend to appear arbitrary stop points toward the long-term goals

• Risk of missing the dates specified in the short-term goals without careful monitoring of compliance

GOALS: MEASURABLE AND MEANINGFUL

In the absence of clear regulatory guidance, therapists are advised to consider both options when establishing goals for individual patients. Clinician decision-making may lead to the use of one model in some situations and the other when the patient condition warrants it.

Writing therapy goals is a complex activity as one tries to balance relevant measurable information with meaningful functionality that incorporates the goals of the patient. When shortcuts are taken, the end result is a set of goals that lack substance and fail to support the need for therapy. Without a clear vision of the outcomes from participation with any of the three therapy disciplines, the decision to end care can be left open to interpretation. As an example, use of "household" as a gait distance can vary greatly depending on the size of the home and can range from the size of a mobile home to a large assisted living complex. Without a measurement, an arbitrary cut off can be set by a third party of 150 feet and care planned that exceeds that could be denied. Again, there is no evidence of distance limitations, but the message is clear: goals must be focused and specific and can be modified over time as the patient progresses through the therapy plan of care.

Planning Care: Putting the Pieces Together

If the assessment provides the foundation and the goals create the vision, then the connection between the two is the plan of care. There are essentially two components to this process: clinical decision-making with respect to the selection of interventions and writing orders for physician signature. Establishing the plan of care requires an analysis of the assessment findings, an understanding of rehabilitation potential, and the ability to put together the most appropriate set of skilled interventions to reach the desired goals. Over time, therapists complete this act without really thinking about all that goes into it and can create plans of care that appear to essentially be the same, regardless of the condition of the patient. This can also happen with setting frequency and duration of care as well as selecting interventions that will be addressed. Support for the medical necessity of physical therapy, occupational therapy, and speech-language pathology requires an effective continuum of information within the documentation of which the plan of care and related orders are critical elements.

Setting Frequency and Duration

Upon completion of the assessment, the therapist must determine the frequency and duration of care. In an ideal world, this decision is driven exclusively by the needs of the patient for skilled services, but there is a very real factor that comes into this process. Many home health agencies are reporting staffing issues to varying degrees for all three therapy disciplines. Even those that appear adequately staffed at the moment will confirm that one vacation or maternity leave can upset the balance and ability to cover patient visits. If the speech therapist is only available to the agency two days a week, it is interesting to note that the established frequency for all of the patients is twice a week. An additional factor is the geography of the service area being covered by the home health agency. Typical staffing patterns reflect more nurses, followed by physical therapists, occupational therapists, and speech-language pathologists in descending order of staff size. This often leaves a smaller group of clinicians trying to cover the entire service area. This leads to visit patterns that are influenced by geography.

As an example, if there are current patients being seen in the same general area that is rather far from the office, new referrals that live in that same direction or area will tend to fall into a similar frequency pattern as a means of managing the schedule. Duration can be influenced by the pressure to continue to take on new patients that can lead to decisions to discharge a patient at a point where he or she is "good enough" as opposed to reaching the highest potential. It is important as professionals to acknowledge the difference between triage and best practice in order to keep the primary focus of frequency and duration the clinical needs of the patient.

Any discussion regarding the setting of frequency and duration for therapy services should include the use of ranges. Common examples are "two to three times per week for four weeks" and "one to two times per week for three to four weeks." First and foremost, it is important to check with the state in which the therapist is practicing to determine if there are any specific restrictions against the use of ranges in physician orders.

In addition, if agency policy does not allow the use of ranges, the staff will be held to the more restrictive standard upon state survey. Once any regulatory issues are cleared, the decision to use or not use ranges must be carefully weighed before moving forward. When ranges are used, the assumption is that the visits will be delivered at the high end at all times and any reduction is based on patient issues alone. Ranges are not intended to accommodate staffing challenges such as therapist illness or vacation. Any decrease in frequency or duration within the range must be documented to show why it occurred. Ranges are expected to be written narrowly such as "one to two times per week for six weeks" as compared to "one to three times per week for four to six weeks." Wider ranges raise questions as to the actual amount of therapy a patient specifically needs. In the second example, it could be anywhere from four to 18 total visits. Based on these types of concerns, many agencies are not allowing the use of ranges. There is nothing inherently wrong with ranges, and those that use them are advised to keep a close watch on how they are being used by nurses and therapists alike.

In the absence of ranges, there can be concerns about compliance with a clearly defined frequency and duration rooted in the risk of providing visits without orders. The "extra visit" delivered based on a scheduling error or the arrival of a piece of equipment must have an attached order or it will not be covered. Impact of this is typically seen more often in relation to duration as therapists have been given a directive to cover the entire 60-day certification period even if they really only plan to see the patient for two weeks. Once again, there is no specific regulation supporting or refuting this process, and if this is set in agency policy there could be issues on state survey if compliance is not consistent. Therapists need to understand why the practice is in place and always keep in mind that the amount of therapy must be defended as medically necessary even if there are orders in place for additional care.

Many agencies utilize the therapy frequency and duration orders to determine the estimated amount the therapy visits for Outcome and Assessment Information Set item M2200 at the start of care for the purposes of projecting payment for the episode. Recent assessment of the accuracy of this projection is less than 25%, which means that the plan of care can and should change over time as patient need dictates. The clinical decision to extend care beyond the original plan or to discontinue earlier than initially expected because the patient no longer needs the skills of a therapist must be supported by written orders for physician signature to confirm his or her involvement in the plan of care.

Orders and Medical Necessity

Every agency has a group of patients that seem to get referred for any and all services by their well-intentioned physicians. Family members can complicate this situation further by requesting orders for therapy despite the fact that there is no reasonable expectation for additional improvement in function. Therapists can find themselves in a difficult position of having a physician order in hand but a lack of clinical support for skilled services. Attempts should be made to explain the situation clearly to the patient, family, and physician. Even if all of these parties insist the care is necessary, it is still the responsibility of the therapist to determine if skilled interventions are warranted. If this cannot be done, then provision of services is not considered covered. If this is a Medicare patient, use of the Home Health Advanced Beneficiary Notice can be an effective and professional way to handle the situation. It outlines in writing that the home health agency is willing to provide specific services to the patient but does not believe that the services will be covered under the Medicare benefit. The agency is informing the patient of the potential costs of the services and asks for a signature to assume financial responsibility should Medicare choose not to pay based on a noncoverage decision. It is interesting to note the ability of this form to change the perspective of the patient and family about what the patient "needs." Communication of any decisions made must include the ordering physician. It is important to be clear that medical necessity will not be supported solely by the presence of a physician's order, but visits can be denied if no order is in place.

485 versus supplemental orders

The level of detail in the orders sent to the physician for signature varies when a therapist completes the admission to the agency compared to when he or she completes the discipline-specific assessment after the case has been opened. Often referred to as the "485," the plan of care generated at the time of admission or recertification is intended to be interdisciplinary and contain a defined set of information about the patient, including but not limited to biographical data, certification dates, physician information, diagnoses, homebound status, activity limitations, as well as frequency, duration, goals, and interventions for all ordered services.

If all assessments occur within the first few days of the episode, then the therapy-specific information should be included in this form and sent for physician signature. If time has lapsed and the 485 has already been completed, then frequency, duration, goals, and interventions are to be sent by each specific therapy to the ordering physician. It is a routine practice to document "eval and treat" on the 485 as a placeholder for therapy services, but additional specific orders will have to be generated and "eval and treat" will not cover a course of physical therapy, occupational therapy, or speech-language pathology.

When utilizing electronic documentation tools, it can be hard to actually see these orders in the literal sense because they can be pulled together from various fields being completed within the system. Therapists should periodically read through the orders being generated as part of the admission process or the discipline-specific assessment to ensure that the necessary and relevant information is being captured in the documentation.

104   The How-to Guide to Home Health Therapy Documentation

Selecting interventions

The clinical decision-making component of establishing a care plan requires more than selecting a few standard items from a list. The three therapy disciplines are often connected to a specific set of patient problems:

- Physical therapy: addresses gait issues

- Occupational therapy: addresses activities of daily living (ADL) and instrumental activities of daily living (IADL) issues

- Speech-language pathology: addresses communication and swallowing issues

Review of records indicates that all three therapies have become quite comfortable, indicating a very similar set of interventions regardless of the status of the patient. Here are the most commonly seen:

- Physical therapy for the following:

  - Gait training

  - Transfer training

  - Balance training

  - Therapeutic exercises

- Occupational therapy for the following:

  - ADL retraining

  - IADL retraining

  - Therapeutic exercises

  - Energy conservation strategies

- Speech-language pathology for the following:

  - Communication strategies

- Oral motor training

- Cognitive retraining

- Memory strategies

Although some of the terminology may differ slightly, the general idea is seen in the listed interventions. Electronic documentation tools often provide these as convenient options that are "point and click" and generate the required information on the 485 or supplemental order without a second thought. Establishing a plan of care that clearly supports the medical necessity of therapy services requires a second look at the words that are being chosen to make sure the level of skill is clear. Here are some examples to consider:

- Mr. Max had a stroke about two weeks ago. His occupational therapist is going to provide "ADL retraining" per the written order. The actual plan is to address bathing issues that are complicated by the tone in his right arm.

- Mrs. Bentley had an exacerbation of heart failure last week. Her occupational therapist is going to provide "ADL retraining" per the written order. The actual plan is to address toileting issues implementing energy conservation strategies due to the dyspnea that limits her ability to perform this task on her own.

- Mr. Stone has mild dementia and was recently started on three new medications. His occupational therapist is going to provide "ADL retraining" per the written order. The actual plan is to instruct him in the use of a pill planner to manage medications safely.

The examples serve the purpose of demonstrating how terms such as "ADL retraining" may not be communicating the level of skilled care being provided by occupational therapy. Similar issues are seen with the intervention of "gait training" because there are actually countless factors that can impact the ability to ambulate and create a patient-specific plan of action. There is nothing specifically incorrect about the interventions being listed in this way, but it may be incomplete when supporting medical necessity. The therapist should look back at the assessment to find the issues identified, especially the "why" behind them, and customize interventions accordingly.

Examples of more detailed interventions for each of the three therapies are as follows. These are not meant to be a new list from which to generate information but to provoke thought about what makes skilled care uniquely physical therapy, occupational therapy, or speech-language pathology.

Physical therapy

+ Gait training focused on balance and strength deficits

+ Gait training incorporating compensatory strategies for visual deficits

+ Transfer training: sit to stand from recliner focused on pain limiting mobility

+ Transfer training: on/off bedside commode focused on lower extremity weakness issues

+ Balance training in standing incorporating leg length discrepancy

+ Balance training in standing focused on vertigo and lower extremity weakness

Occupational therapy

+ ADL retraining: bathing inclusive of fear issue due to recent fall

+ ADL retraining: lower body dressing using adaptive equipment

+ ADL retraining: grooming with focus on cognitive limitations

+ IADL retraining: laundry management incorporating use of new walker

+ IADL retraining: meal preparation using microwave following multiple-step commands

+ Energy conservation: pursed lip breathing during bathing activities

Speech-language pathology

+ Communication strategies: focus on ability to communicate basic needs to caregivers

+ Oral motor training: focus on tongue coordination

+ Oral motor training: focus on improving the quality of the swallow

+ Cognitive retraining: establish a drug diary for medication management

+ Cognitive retraining: focus on moving to mastery of multiple step commands

+ Memory strategies: instruct in use of calendar to track appointments

Beyond the areas traditionally considered to be therapy related, a comprehensive care plan may also address interfering pain, pressure ulcer risk, as well as management of incontinence and skin integrity. It is important to keep in mind that each individual service is one piece of the overall care plan for the patient. The most effective plans of care keep the patient at the center and are truly interdisciplinary, utilizing the full scope of skills available as a coordinated team.

At the mention of the need for additional detail in therapy documentation, concerns are often raised about the amount of information required as well as the time consumption involved. The examples provided illustrate that it is not going to require multiple paragraphs to increase the ability to communicate the complexity of therapy interventions. It requires a renewed focus on what skilled therapy really consists of and to empower individual therapists to take credit for the care they provide to people in need.

108   The How-to Guide to Home Health Therapy Documentation

Routine Visits: The Need for Ongoing Therapy

When looking at a comprehensive set of therapy documentation, from the initial assessment to the ultimate discharge, there are certain time points that tend to reflect a higher level of content when compared to others. Assessments by design facilitate detail in support of skilled activities being done on that visit. The same is generally true for therapy visits that are connected to the completion of the Outcome and Assessment Information Set, such as the discharge from the agency. The breakdown in content that impacts the ability of the therapist to support medical necessity is more often seen on the routine follow-up visit. Documentation can slip almost imperceptibly into repetitive information and lack clarity around the need for a skilled therapist to continue working with the patient. Therapists are challenged to maintain a consistent focus on what constitutes skilled care and ensure that the quality of documentation is consistent throughout the episode.

Continuity

When assessing the visit patterns of clinicians practicing in home health, all three therapy disciplines tend to have a higher level of continuity when compared to nursing. In many cases, it may only be one or two individual physical therapists, occupational therapists, or speech-language pathologists working with the patient. Based on caseload demands, it is not unheard of for a patient to interact with five different nurses over the course of two weeks of care. The risk involved with this level of continuity is complacency with respect to documentation content. When there is a high likelihood of the therapist making most if not all of the subsequent visits, it is quite easy to miss aspects of documentation and read between the lines when reviewing the notes because he or she knows the patient situation very well. As the total number of therapy visits increases, the quality of documentation content tends to decrease. Taking into consideration the perception of some that therapy practice in home health has been influenced by the reimbursement structure of the prospective payment system calls the need for a higher number of therapy visits into question. Combining this concern with the aforementioned decline in the quality of documentation content over time can be a recipe for denial. No one is suggesting that putting more therapists in the mix to decrease continuity is a viable solution as this would be disruptive to patients and therapists alike and would not guarantee an improvement in the level of detail being documented. The issue raised is the need to remain focused on supporting the medical necessity of every therapy visit from the first one to the last.

Defining Intervention

It is interesting to note how often the term "intervention" is used when developing care plans and supporting medical necessity on follow-up visits, but do we really understand what it means? As with the word "necessity," additional insights can be gained by looking at the actual definition of the term. According to the *Merriam-Webster's Medical Dictionary*, intervention is "the act or fact or a method of interfering with the outcome or course especially of a condition or process (as to prevent harm or improve intervention) (*http://dictionary.reference.com/browse/interventionfunctioning*).

It is doubtful that any therapist has thought about the care being provided as "interfering," but that component is at the core of supporting skill. The provision of therapy requires active participation of the patient and the therapist. In addition, the therapist must document clearly how his or her activities as uniquely one of the three therapies and could not have been done by someone else with the same results. Therapists generally do a good job demonstrating what the patient was doing during a visit but often leave themselves out of the picture. This is evident in the prevalence of statements similar to these seen in records:

+ "Patient completed bathing activity"

+ "Patient demonstrated dressing with adaptive equipment"

+ "Patient progressed ambulation to 50 feet with walker"

+ "Patient did home exercise program (HEP)"

When seen in print, the terms "completed," "demonstrated," "progressed," and "did" clearly indicate what the patient is doing during the activity but have no information as to what the therapist is doing other than recording observations. As with assessments, therapists paid more attention to what specifically they were doing with the patients when we were learning our skills. We were concerned about doing the best possible job and not missing anything. Practice has increased in breadth and depth over time and with experience to the point where interventions are simply an extension of who we are without even thinking about it. Calling what the therapist does on a visit "gait training," "activities of daily living (ADL) retraining," or "oral motor training" is not enough detail as those are more categories than specifics indicative of skilled care. The challenge is to step out of old habits that may have been accepted at other points in our careers and plot a new course to show the value of therapy throughout an episode of care.

Therapeutic Exercises

A great example of both the lack of necessary detail as well as the opportunity to impact the quality of documentation content is in the area of therapeutic exercise. Establishing an exercise program is a routine activity for all three of the therapies and includes the need for teaching the patient and/or caregiver how to follow through correctly. Documentation of exercise is often viewed as tedious and redundant, with the primary focus being on listing the names and the number of repetitions associated with each. There are times that the level of detail is even less with statements such as "seated exercises × 10 reps," "standing exercises at sink × 15 reps," and "oral motor exercises × 10 reps." It can become even more problematic when "see exercises from last visit" is used as a shortcut. Although it is important to speak to the exercises themselves, there is a critical element missing. Think about what a therapist is actually doing while exercises are being performed. If it is just counting, the need for skilled intervention is in question. Here are some examples.

- The physical therapist initiated standing hip abduction and hip extension exercises bilaterally as well as partial squats with Mr. Anderson on the third visit. Because this was new information, she had to demonstrate each of the exercises and provide continuous verbal cues to ensure proper performance. She is confident he understood the instruction and left him with pictures to help him remember how to complete the exercises correctly. Her note indicates "the patient completed standing exercises at the counter × 10 reps each." On the next visit, Mr. Anderson proudly tells the physical therapist how well he did with his exercises but when he starts to demonstrate, there are issues with his performance. He is not completing the full range of motion (ROM) and tends to lean excessively during the hip exercises but does well with the squats. The therapist demonstrates the other two exercises again and this time the patient requires verbal cueing about 50% of the task. On this visit, the therapist documents "the patient completed standing exercises at the counter × 10 reps each." Some may focus on the fact that the three exercises should have been listed, and they have a point. The larger issues are that neither sample of the documentation reflects the demonstration or verbal cues provided by the therapist or how those changed between the two visits—both of which are the components that actually show skilled care.

- The occupational therapist instructed Mrs. Bond in an upper extremity (UE) exercise program using red theraband on the second visit, which is on a Friday. Written instructions including pictures are reviewed and, with a few cues, Mrs. Bond is pleased with how well she can complete 10 repetitions. The therapist documents "patient performed UE ther ex with red theraband × 10 reps bilaterally." On Monday, Mrs. Bond's granddaughter is present for the visit and reports that the patient did so well she had her do 15 repetitions without any increase in pain. When the therapist asks Mrs. Bond to demonstrate her program, he is very concerned that she is not anchoring the theraband correctly and not completing the full active ROM (AROM) as instructed. He asks the patient to find the pictures that were left and goes over each exercise again step by step, including the granddaughter in the education. By the end of the visit, the occupational therapist is confident they will be able to complete the exercises correctly but wants to check again on the next visit. For this visit, the therapist documents "patient performed UE ther ex with red theraband × 15 reps bilaterally." Although there is an increase in repetitions, there is no mention of the quality of performance or the skilled teaching provided by the therapist. In this example, the granddaughter was able to increase repetitions but did not notice the issues with technique. If progress with therapeutic exercises is only measured by repetitions, then there is no need for the occupational therapist to address these because the family member can handle that without skilled intervention.

- The speech-language pathologist completes her assessment and, based on the findings, initiates an oral motor exercise program for Mr. Caldwell. She instructs him to perform these in front of a mirror to make sure he is doing them correctly and has his wife observe the session to provide reinforcement. Mr. Caldwell was recently diagnosed with dementia and has had some issues remembering new information. The therapist documents "patient instructed in oral motor exercises." On the next visit, the therapist notices that the mirror she had placed on the table was absent. When asked about it, the patient's wife reports "it was in the way so I moved it." After setting the mirror in place, the therapist asks the patient to complete the exercises. She is pleased he is able to do them very well with respect to basic technique, but he hurries and does not complete the number of repetitions he is supposed to. The therapist reminds him to slow down and take his time. He reports, "I'm fine. I don't like these. Why do I have to do them?" The speech-language pathologist explains the purpose behind these exercises and how doing them will improve his ability to communicate clearly. He agrees they are a good idea and slows down his performance. The therapist speaks with his wife about how the exercises should be performed as well. She documents "patient completed oral motor exercises." Not only is there a lack of detail as to the specific exercises and repetitions in the example, but the instruction provided is not captured at all. If the patient can "complete" these without any issues noted then on future visits the need for a therapist to continue to observe him do these is not well supported.

Although inclusion of some form of exercise program is expected as part of a therapy plan of care, documentation connected to follow-up visits often omits the details that would confirm that the intervention requires the skills of the therapist. The absence of information creates the impression that anyone can provide the same level of care. It is imperative for therapists to not assume that documenting the name of an exercise along with the number of repetitions implies the complex level of skill that is actually involved in the provision of a therapeutic exercise program.

Therapy and "Training"

The plan of care sets the expectation of what will be addressed over the course of therapy. As mentioned previously, the word "training" appears very often in therapy documentation. Nursing has its own version of the same issue in the word "teaching." It appears that clinicians are visiting patients and training, training, and training or teaching, teaching, and teaching over and over again until the discharge visit. At that time, the patient suddenly learns everything and no longer needs training or teaching. No one is saying the word itself is the issue, but it must be kept in the proper context. "Gait training," "ADL retraining," and "cognitive training" are not clearly defined terms but should be seen as category headings requiring additional patient-specific details. This is an extension of the discussion in the chapter on assessment in that there needs to be a connection to the specific deficits that are being addressed during the task.

- Mr. Dodds has Parkinson's disease. During gait training, the physical therapist assistant has to cue him to take longer steps when using his walker and to be careful when moving from the linoleum to carpeting. The therapist documents, "gait training: patient ambulated 75 feet × 1 with walker and stand-by assist (SBA)."

  - Better option: Gait training: patient ambulated 75 × 1 with walker and SBA. He consistently requires verbal cues regarding step length and when transitioning surfaces.

- Mrs. Easton has heart failure and becomes SOB when walking more than 20 feet. During gait training, the physical therapist assistant coaches her to perform her pursed lip breathing when walking as well as to slow down her pace as she tends to hurry. The therapist documents, "Gait training: patient ambulated 75 feet × 1 with walker and SBA.

  - Better option: gait training: patient ambulated 75 feet × 1 with walker and SBA. She requires verbal cues to slow pace and was instructed in use of pursed lip breathing when SOB; 100% verbal cues needed for consistent follow-through.

- Mr. Finnegan had his hip replaced about two weeks ago and is anxious when putting weight on his right leg. During gait training, the physical therapist assistant encourages him to not stay up on his toes on the right foot anymore because his weight-bearing restriction was lifted. He is hesitant to try but after the first few feet he is able to put his foot down flat but is still not putting much weight through it. The therapist documents, "gait training: patient ambulated 75 feet × 1 with walker and SBA."

  - Better option: gait training: patient ambulated 75 feet × 1 with walker and SBA. He requires consistent verbal cues for correct foot positioning on the right due to anxiety about recent change in weight-bearing status.

Training implies action. Suppose you decided to work with a personal trainer to meet your goals for an upcoming beach season. The trainer arrives and takes a seat on your sofa and begins to take notes. He asks you to demonstrate the exercises you have been doing up to this point and has no comments as you complete them. He tells you what a good job you did and proceeds to schedule the next appointment. Would you pay for this service? What is missing? The involvement of a trainer creates the expectation that he or she is going to do something that adds value to your current activity program. Critiquing performance, offering suggestions, adding new exercises, and pushing the program to new levels are implied in the word "trainer." If you could achieve the same results without the trainer then you would not want to pay for this service. The goals would not be reached with passive observation alone and without the appropriate level of detail it is the same impression given by therapy documentation. Every visit must clearly show that what the therapist is contributing could not have been done by another discipline or a nonskilled caregiver.

Examples of Necessary Care

Examples of more detailed interventions for each of the three therapies are as follows. A single statement does not support medical necessity alone and must be integrated with other statements to create the picture of the care provided to the patient. These examples are not meant to be a list from which to generate information but to provoke thought about what makes skilled care uniquely physical therapy, occupational therapy, or speech-language pathology, specifically addressing unique patient issues.

Physical therapy

- Gait training: include more than distance, device, and level of assistance

  - Patient ambulated 50 feet with walker and minimal assistance due to weakness in left lower extremity and complaints of mild vertigo. Verbal cues required for 50% of the task for proper sequencing with the walker.

  - Patient ambulated 85 feet with cane and supervision on level surfaces and 25% verbal cues regarding cane placement. On grass in back yard, assistance increased to contact guard assist (CGA) and verbal cues to 50% due to increased unsteadiness and distance decreased to 45 feet before rest break is needed.

- Transfer training: consider the components of each specific transfer

  - Patient required minimal assistance to scoot forward in her chair. Once in that position, she required SBA to complete a sit to stand transfer.

  - Patient instructed in pushing up from his chair using the armrests when coming to stand. He requires 100% verbal cues for this component due to limited attention span.

- Bed mobility training: outline challenges to specific aspects

  - Patient rolls to right with minimal assistance to reach railing due to pain limiting her ability to reach. Instructed her to lower how far she attempts to reach to decrease level of pain during task.

  - Patient instructed in bridging to decrease the amount of assistance the caregiver has to provide during hygiene. Patient able to bridge with minimal assistance once feet are in place.

- Fall risk reduction: connect specific risks to need for physical therapy

  - Instructed patient and daughter to not use a step stool for reaching higher shelves due to recent fall.

  - Patient wearing socks when ambulating and noted to slip slightly on the kitchen floor twice during gait training. Recommended the use of grip socks or nonskid slippers to reduce fall risk and patient agreeable. Will monitor for follow through on subsequent visits.

- Self-care training: ability to ambulate and transfer should connect to functional tasks

  - Patient ambulated 60 feet × 1 with rolling walker and minimal assistance that increased to moderate assistance when going through doorway to access bathroom

  - Patient ambulated up five steps to access her bedroom on second floor using railing and SBA due to fatigue after first two steps

- Balance training: consider tests and movement beyond "poor, fair, good"

  - Single leg stance: left = 20 seconds, right = 32 seconds

  - Unsupported stance with eyes closed = 10 seconds with moderate increase in sway noted

ROUTINE VISITS: THE NEED FOR ONGOING THERAPY

+ Strength training: include the role of the therapist

    – Seated exercises: 10 reps each of hip flexion, knee extension, and ankle pumps bilaterally with 50% verbal cues to complete full AROM

    – Standing exercises: 15 squats at counter with CGA due to increased unsteadiness as repetitions increase

+ Muscle tone: consider connection of tone to activity

    – Weight bearing through left hand on the armrest to assist with sit to stand transfer equalizes tone and increases ability to assist

    – Weight shift in standing at counter with minimal assistance to right increasing weight bearing to decrease extensor tone in right leg

+ ROM: include the role of the therapist

    – AROM of right knee extension × 10 repetitions with minimal assistance to achieve neutral

    – Self-assisted passive ROM (PROM) for left shoulder flexion × 10 reps with 75% verbal cues for correct technique

+ Endurance training: utilize dyspnea as indicated and connect to functional task

    – Progressing time patient can sustain ambulation this visit to three minutes before becoming SOB in preparation for cardiac rehabilitation

    – Standing at side of bed for two minutes with minimal assistance × 2 with walker as pre-gait activity

+ Edema management: include circumferential measurements, descriptors, and functional impact

    – Upon arrival, noted that footrest was not near the patient's chair. It appears she has not been using it as instructed and reviewed need to do so to decrease swelling in bilateral feet.

- During ambulation noted that compression socks were not being worn. Patient's daughter reports they are being washed and she will put them back on this afternoon.

- Cognitive/behavioral: consider impact of plan of care

  - HEP instruction provided in picture format due to patient's inability to read

  - Treatment session limited to 30 minutes as patient became anxious about visit to doctor later today

- Communication/comprehension: consider impact of education

  - HEP instruction must be in written format for appropriate follow-through due to limited verbal comprehension.

  - Patient initiated use of communication board without reminders to tell therapist she wanted a drink. This was first instance of this noted with physical therapist indicating carryover of speech-language pathology instruction.

- Environment: focus on what is unique to the patient situation

  - Fatigue with ambulation is increased when on plush carpet in family room.

  - Patient requires minimal assistance with transfer from recliner chair due to low seat height. Patient unwilling to use a different chair or modify height of current chair.

- Safety awareness: determine what makes the task or activity "safe" or "unsafe"

  - Patient able to recall two of three hip precautions independently, and verbal cues needed for no flexion past 90 degrees

  - Patient requires verbal cues throughout tub transfer to maintain non–weight bearing status of right lower extremity

- Vision: consider impact on function and plan of care

    - Patient requires verbal cues to check for obstacles on the right side while ambulating due to limited peripheral vision in his right eye

    - HEP information converted to large print due to limited vision and improve carryover

- Sensation: screen for problems that impact function as well as other issues

    - Instructed patient to visualize foot placement on stairs carefully due to peripheral neuropathy.

    - Patient required verbal reminder to inspect her feet after gait training with new slippers to check for any areas of pressure. She is a diabetic with decreased sensation in both feet.

Occupational therapy

ADLs retraining: focus on "why" the specific level of assistance is needed. ADLs include but are not limited to:

- Grooming

    - Patient completed shaving with supervision and verbal cues to complete multiple-step commands

    - Patient requires minimal assistance to maintain balance while standing to brush hair

- Dressing

    - Once clothing was handed to patient, minimal assistance needed to put on shirt due to left shoulder pain

    - Patient requires moderate assistance with donning/doffing compression stocking due to decreased grip strength in left hand

- Bathing

    - Instructed patient in correct placement of transfer bench and grab bars in preparation for shower training next week

- Patient requires maximum assistance with set up for sponge bathing and CGA during the task due to development of dyspnea after four minutes of activity

+ Toileting hygiene

- Instructed the caregiver in how to support patient when leaning forward and provide minimal verbal cues to ensure perineal hygiene is completed thoroughly

- Patient is able to use a dressing stick to pull up pants after using the toilet with SBA and occasional verbal cue for proper technique

+ Medication management

- Practiced opening medication bottles with patient who was able to complete task one of three attempts.

- Pill planner color coded and guide created to assist patient with keeping a.m. and p.m. medications separated correctly. Practiced using the guide with 50% verbal cues needed at this time.

+ Feeding

- A nonskid placemat provided to patient, and with the plate secured, she is able to feed herself independently.

- Adapted spoon trialed with patient but did not improve his ability to feed himself. Will trial again in one week to allow strength to improve.

Instrumental ADLs (IADL) retraining: focus on "why" the specific level of assistance is needed. IADLs include but are not limited to:

+ Meal preparation

- Walker tray delivered to patient over the weekend and attached by occupational therapist assistant correctly. Demonstrated to patient how to arrange items for transport in the kitchen. Currently, she is not independent and will require supervision and occasional verbal cues to reinforce safe performance.

- Discussed purchase of microwave with patient's son as use of stove is currently unsafe due to leaving burners on if alone.

+ Money management

- Patient instructed how to organize incoming bills with colored files to improve ability to manage them herself. Currently, she requires supervision with this task.

- Patient now able to write with adapted pen independently. Applied this skill to simulated check writing and increased difficulty staying on specific lines due to visual issues. Provided additional simulated checks for patient to practice prior to next occupational therapy visit.

+ Household management

- Patient is currently dependent with laundry. Demonstrated the option of using a rolling basket to transport clothes and patient able to return demo with SBA for balance.

- Dishes arranged in cabinets to lower those used most often to within reach. Once completed, patient able to safely access dishes independently.

+ Functional mobility training: address mobility impact on ADLs and IADLs

- Reinforced use of walker when ambulating into bathroom for grooming activities

- Notes patient tends to leave her walker by the counter during meal preparation with increased unsteadiness when carrying items from the refrigerator to the stove

+ Transfers training: consider the components of each specific transfer

- Patient completed shower transfer with reminders to use the grab bars and supervision.

- Patient requires supervision when using the transfer bench due to memory issues with proper sequence. Instructed daughter how to assist patient and return demo confirms understanding of technique.

+ Bed mobility training: outline challenges to specific aspects

    − Patient rolls to right with minimal assistance to reach railing due to pain limiting her ability to reach. Instructed her to lower how far she attempts to reach to decrease level of pain during task.

    − Patient instructed in bridging to decrease the amount of assistance the caregiver has to provide during hygiene. Patient able to bridge with minimal assistance once feet are in place.

+ Fall risk reduction: connect specific risks to need for occupational therapy

    − Instructed patient to remove throw rugs from the bathroom as walker gets caught on them during toileting. Patient verbalized understanding and will confirm follow-through on next visit.

    − Observation of dressing raises concerns over patient leaning too far over and leaning on the nightstand. Instructed patient in appropriate dressing technique using a reacher. Patient requires maximum verbal cues to complete.

+ Balance training: consider tests and movement beyond "poor, fair, good" while connecting issues to function.

    − Reaching for objects outside base of support in sitting requires moderate assistance due to patient anxiety

    − Static sitting at edge of bed requires CGA and tolerance is three minutes before pain limits continuation

+ Strength training: include the role of the therapist

    − Added 2 pounds weight to shoulder flexion, abduction, and extension and decreased repetitions to 10 with supervision to ensure full ROM is completed

    − Review of HEP indicates patient is able to complete four of five exercises independently but requires verbal cues and demonstration to correctly complete full range of shoulder external rotation

- Muscle tone: consider connection of tone to activity

  – Instructed caregiver in proper application of splint for right hand to decrease flexor tone in preparation for specific ADL tasks

  – Patient requires maximum verbal cues to correctly complete stretching of right wrist as tone management strategy

- ROM: include the role of the therapist

  – AROM of right elbow extension × 10 repetitions with minimal assistance to achieve neutral

  – Self-assisted PROM for left shoulder abduction × 10 reps with 75% verbal cues for correct technique

- Endurance training: utilize dyspnea as indicated and connect to functional task

  – Patient able to complete bathing with CGA requiring rest break after four minutes due to dyspnea

  – Patient requires a seated rest break of three minutes during meal preparation after completing 10 minutes of activity in standing

- Edema: include circumferential measurements, descriptors, and functional impact

  – Upon arrival, noted that footrest was not near the patient's chair. It appears she has not been using it as instructed and reviewed need to do so to decrease swelling in bilateral feet.

  – During dressing noted that compression socks were not being worn. Patient's daughter reports they are being washed and she will put them back on this afternoon.

- Cognition/communication/comprehension/psychosocial issues: connect concerns to functional tasks

  – Patient requires 50% verbal cues to complete a five-step set of directions to reheat a meal.

– Patient's HEP instructions provided in written form due to limited ability to comprehend verbal information. Patient able to return demo independently the three exercises communicated in this way and will confirm this strategy with the interdisciplinary team.

+ Environment: focus on what is unique to the patient situation

– Proximity of toilet to vanity prohibits use of commode frame, so training will utilize a raised toilet seat. Patient performs toilet transfer with supervision post setup and instruction.

– Flooring in kitchen is uneven and impacts ability to smoothly roll a walker. Nonslip placemat added to walker tray to decrease slippage of items, and patient instructed to utilize during meal preparation activities. Verbalized understanding this visit.

+ Safety: determine what makes the task or activity "safe" or "unsafe"

– Patient requires supervision during meal preparation due to impulsivity. Instructed caregiver how to verbal cue patient regarding pacing. Will need to reinforce compliance on next several visits.

– Patient insisting on using a wooden board on his walker to transport items; the board is not stable for larger items. Discussed trial with walker basket and he is willing to try this on next visit.

+ Sensorimotor: connect issues to functional tasks

– Instructed patient's new caregiver to increase volume when speaking with patient as he is not confused but is hard of hearing.

– Patient requires minimal assistance during setup of medications due to vision limitations due to moderate macular degeneration. Compensatory strategies require 100% verbal cues to complete correctly at this time.

Speech therapy

- Oral motor function: strength, ROM, sensation, and function

  - Patient requires verbal cues 50% of the time with oral motor exercises involving his tongue for correct technique.

  - Instructed patient on pacing breathing while speaking to manage impact of dyspnea. After demonstration of technique, patient able to return demo with minimal verbal cues.

- Swallowing: posture, positioning, consistencies, and diet

  - Instructed caregiver in correct amount of thickener to achieve nectar consistency for beverages. Caregiver anxiety about this task leads to errors when he does not follow written instructions. Discussed the need to relax and make sure the instructions are followed. Will need reinforcement on subsequent visits to confirm consistent follow-through.

  - Patient requires minimal assistance to achieve appropriate sitting posture when eating. As task progresses, verbal cues required to maintain position due to increasing fatigue.

- Cognition/communication: attention, orientation, recall, and memory

  - Instructed patient's daughter to turn off the television during meals to increase patient's ability to focus on swallowing technique due to current level of distractibility and increasing risk of aspiration

  - Patient provided with large print calendar and with 100% verbal cues was able to write down home care appointments for the following week

- Speech/language: articulation, comprehension, hearing, and expression

  - Patient requires moderate verbal cues to decrease pace of verbal communication to improve ability to articulate clearly. Instructed caregiver in proper cueing for carryover until next visit.

  - Recommend visit to audiologist to assess effectiveness of current hearing aids. A dry erase board provided to the patient and a sign posted to inform caregivers to write down information if patient is unable to hear them clearly.

Fundamental Question

Novice and seasoned therapists can struggle to integrate themselves into their documentation on every visit, yet it is those aspects that support the medical necessity of the care provided. To gain the proper perspective, consider the following question while exiting the patient's home after the visit: What did I contribute that is unique to my discipline and indispensable to this particular patient?

Reassessments: Home Health Requirements

Assessments create the foundation for the plan of care, and reassessments serve the purpose of periodic inspections to make sure the building of the plan is going smoothly. The concept of reviewing the plan of care and determining whether modifications need to be made is not an idea created by Medicare or specific to home health. In many therapy textbooks and published guidelines for practice, assessment and reassessment are presented together as a unified concept. The component that is not defined in a universal standard is when reassessments should occur. This is where state practice acts and third-party payers such as Medicare may step in and set time frames for any or all settings in which therapists practice. For home health, there are really two different mechanisms in place for formal review of the plan of care: recertification and reassessment. Both of these have documentation expectations that are rooted in the need to confirm the medical necessity of the care being provided and, if not clearly met, risk the denial of payment for services rendered.

Recertification

The Home Health Prospective Payment System (PPS) is built on a 60-day episode model. The start of care (SOC) date initiates the episode, and the comprehensive assessment drives the plan of care that is established at the onset of services. The original plan, as well as any supplemental orders, is only effective within that single certification period. As calendar day 60 approaches, disciplines anticipating the need to continue care beyond that point need to discuss this as a team and determine which one of them will complete the mandatory recertification Outcome and Assessment Information Set (OASIS) within the last five days of the episode. It is true that only one clinician fills in the actual OASIS form, but as discussed in the chapter on OASIS, it is the responsibility of the interdisciplinary team to collaborate and ensure accurate data is collected.

The task of completing a recertification OASIS can be done by a registered nurse, a physical therapist, an occupational therapist, or a speech-language pathologist. Unlike the SOC OASIS, there is no regulation with respect to which one of these services has to be the one to complete the document. It is up to the agency and the team to decide. In addition to the OASIS itself, additional assessment items are completed very similarly to the content of the initial assessment done on admission. The purpose of collecting data again is to determine any measurable impact of the care provided up to this time point. At this time, the plan of care must also be created for the new 60-day period. The expectation is for the current plan to be reviewed and updated as indicated based on assessment findings and necessary changes to frequency, duration, interventions, and goals. There are times that the clinical findings support the decision to continue the original plan of care into the next certification period, but careful attention must be paid to confirm that is the best course of action for the patient. Clinical judgment and critical thinking skills are necessary to validate the medical necessity of continued care. Measurable and meaningful changes to the plan of care that correlate to the clinical findings support the need for skilled services to continue to be involved with the patient.

Although one discipline completes the recertification OASIS and is responsible for updating the formal plan of care, any additional discipline expecting to continue care into the next certification period has to demonstrate the components of a recertification process in the documentation. These include but are not limited to:

+ Objective measurements to demonstrate changes in the patient as a result of care already provided

+ Review of current frequency and duration with adjustments as necessary

+ Review of interventions showing which ones need to continue and which can be discontinued

+ Updated goals based on progress to date with removal of those that are no longer applicable

+ Summary of progress to date and impact of care to this point as well as why additional services would be of benefit to this patient

The mandatory recertification every 60 days is the mechanism for periodic formal justification for services to continue. The intent is to prevent care plans that go on with no end in sight and make clinicians accountable for documenting the need for skilled care at defined intervals.

128   The How-to Guide to Home Health Therapy Documentation

Therapy Reassessments

Although the recertification process applies to all home health services that plan to continue into another 60-day episode, mandatory reassessment is a specific requirement for therapy services that began in 2011. Practice patterns suggest that there are not a large number of patients that have therapy active at the time of recertification as most therapy care plans begin and end within a single certification period. In those situations, there is no requirement in place to address when a therapy plan should be reviewed and updated.

Without any requirements, the expectation was that therapists would complete this periodically and voluntarily to document support of the medical necessity of their services. Review of documentation does not appear to confirm that this activity was being completed with any regularity, even at time points where the expectation for this type of assessment would be more obvious. Consider a case in which a patient is evaluated by the speech-language pathologist and the plan of care includes a frequency and duration of "two times a week for four weeks." Initial goals and interventions are determined and care delivery begins. Near the end of the fourth week, a new order appears that reads "continue to week two" with the same interventions listed as they were on the original order. In order to create this new order, one would assume that on one of the visits made during the fourth week the speech-language pathologist determined that additional care was needed. It could be that progress was slower than expected, there may have been cancelled visits that delayed attainment of goals, or that progress was better than expected and new goals are being set. Something clinically driven led to the decision to extend care, yet far too often little to no detail is documented. The visits in week four look like the ones completed in week three. Week five begins with no clear reason, and visits progress as though this was the original plan.

This may not impact the level of skilled care provided to the patient, but the lack of documentation puts the medical necessity at risk. It is important to understand that the perception of payer sources leans toward the idea that because more total therapy visits triggers more revenue, the lack of clinical justification for continued care can be interpreted as being driven more by financial implications than patient need. Medicare is specifically interested when the total number of therapy visits within a certification period reaches 14 to 19 as well as 20 or more because those two points in the reimbursement continuum have the potential to add even more money to the episodic payment. In response to the lack of clarity and concerns regarding perceived incentives in the payment methodology, the mandatory model for therapy reassessments was implemented impacting episodes that began on or after April 1, 2011.

Who is responsible?

The task of completing the therapy reassessment falls to what Medicare calls the "qualified therapist" and not to the therapist assistant. The reasoning is that the skill set required to review the plan of care and to make changes based on clinical findings is in the scope of practice for the physical therapist, occupational therapist, and speech-language pathologist. Completion of the reassessment requires the qualified therapist to make a visit to the home and should be incorporated into a treatment visit already planned for the patient. The reassessment requirement is not related in any way to supervisory visits for therapist assistants. It is in effect for all home health agencies, including those that do not utilize assistants. Currently, the requirements are for Medicare fee-for-service patients but monitoring of expectations of other payment programs going forward will be important to ensure compliance.

Components of reassessment

In order to understand the documentation expectation of a therapy reassessment, clarity as to the focus of this task is pivotal. Use of the word "assessment" triggers a response from therapists that a complete new evaluation is required and for some the concern that an OASIS form is somehow connected to this time point—but neither of these concepts are accurate. The fundamental intent is to reevaluate the plan of care to confirm that the skilled therapy services continue to be warranted and making changes as needed based on objective clinical information.

Here are the key pieces of information that must be clear in the documentation of a therapy reassessment visit:

1. **Objective assessments:** The data collected should relate back to the previous assessment to show measurable changes in the patient. Compliance does not mandate that this include any specific named tools but sequential measurements are important to quantify changes in the patient's functional status.

2. **Expectation of progress:** There needs to be a clinically supported statement that the patient will continue to demonstrate meaningful progress or will resume progress after a plateau or regression. If progress has not been seen at the time of the reassessment but is expected as a result of additional therapy, the services are considered skilled care. There is nothing stating that if there has not been progress discharge is required immediately. The inclusion of the word "plateau" is very significant as it has long been rumored in home health that lack of progress over three visits (or some other randomly selected number) confirms plateau and therapy must end services. The language of PPS 2011 reinforces that there must be positive impact from therapy interventions, but defining skill also involves what the therapist is contributing that will lead to progress at a later point.

3. **Support for effectiveness of therapy:** Effectiveness is an interesting word choice as it will not be enough to state "continue skilled physical therapy per plan of care." By definition, effectiveness is "producing a decided, decisive, claimed, or desired effect." Once again, therapists need to take credit for the complexity of care being provided from the first visit onward and how those specific interventions are impacting the patient in a meaningful way.

4. **Plan to continue or discontinue services:** If the clinical findings and the professional judgment of the therapist support a decision to continue or discontinue, the frequency and duration will be impacted accordingly.

5. **New orders as indicated:** When changes to the plan of care are initiated, new orders for physician signature are to be generated in accordance with current regulations and agency policies.

For purposes of tracking compliance, many agencies utilize a specific documentation form for the reassessment visits. Although there is no formal requirement for this, effectiveness does allow for documentation triggers to be created to ensure that the key components are present in the content.

When are reassessments required?

Most therapists can agree that performing reassessments is really not a new concept and that the content requirements are not excessive to demonstrate ongoing medical necessity. The issue causing more frustration is the required time points at which they must be completed. There are three key points that must be addressed: minimally every 30 days and the 13th and 19th therapy visit. To be clear, there is nothing clinically relevant about therapy visit numbers 13 or 19. The selection of those two visit numbers are not random but are directly connected to Medicare home health payment methodology because visit numbers 14 and 20 carry additional reimbursement implications beyond the revenue related to the visit number itself.

In order to navigate how these reassessments will be scheduled, two concepts have to exist simultaneously:

1. The counting of therapy visits in the Medicare payment model is always a cumulative number of completed physical therapy, occupational therapy, and speech-language pathology visits within each individual 60-day episode. With respect to "minimally" every 30 days, the first therapy evaluation begins the calendar day counting. Only billable visits are counted and, to ensure an accurate count, missed or cancelled visits must be removed from any counting process.

2. The act of completing the reassessment must be done by any active therapy discipline separately. It is not within the scope of practice of one therapy to determine effectiveness and update the plan of care for another. That responsibility falls to each therapy specifically. As an example, the physical therapist can and should include information in the documentation that generally supports the need for occupational therapy services but cannot be responsible to create or update the plan of care—frequency/duration, interventions, and goals—specific to that discipline.

Once these two concepts are understood, the scheduling of reassessments must figure out how to be compliant with both of them in cases with one therapy in contrast to those with multiple therapies providing care.

Single therapy involved

+ **Minimally every 30 days:** If the frequency and duration result in reaching 30 calendar days from the previous therapy assessment prior to visit number 13, the reassessment is due prior to day 30. There is no definition or time window for "minimally" so this can be scheduled for week two or three of care when anticipating reaching the 30-day requirement. Waiting until the last minute can create situations where reassessment visits are very close together or a patient cancellation risks compliance. When a reassessment is completed, the 30-day calendar is reset, and the date of that visit is the starting point.

- **Example 1:** The physical therapy plan of care is two week six. A reassessment is anticipated at the end of the fourth week, but the therapist knows the patient will be unavailable that week due to planned medical tests. The therapist schedules to complete it during week three at the same time as the supervisory visit for the physical therapy assistant.

- **Example 2:** The speech-language pathology plan of care is three week five. The therapist is aware that 30 days will be reached before the 13th visit so plans to reassess the patient at the end of week two and again on visit 13 expected during week five.

- **13th therapy visit:** A reassessment is due on the literal 13th visit. If the patient resides in a rural area (as designated by core-based statistical area [CBSA] code), the visit can occur on visit 11, 12, or 13.

  - **Example 3a:** The occupational therapist plans a total of 15 visits. After addressing the implications of minimally every 30 days, she plans to complete the reassessment on Friday's visit, which is number 13.

  - **Example 3b:** The therapist learns that the patient in example 3a resides in a rural area. She can schedule the reassessment on visit number 11, which simultaneously complies with minimally every 30 days.

- **19th therapy visit:** A reassessment is due on the literal 19th visit. If the patient resides in a rural area (as designated by CBSA code), the visit can occur on visit 17, 18, or 19.

  - **Example 4a:** The physical therapist plans a total of 23 visits. After addressing the implications of minimally every 30 days and the 13th visit, he plans to complete the reassessment on Friday's visit, which is number 19.

  - **Example 4b:** The therapist learns that the patient in example 4a resides in a rural area. He can schedule the upcoming reassessment on visit number 18 and complete the supervisory visit for the assistant at the same time.

♦ **Patient-driven exception:** If it is anticipated that the literal 13th or 19th visit cannot be made for a patient-driven reason, the reassessment can be completed in the same window as for rural patients and still be compliant.

Multiple therapies involved

♦ **Minimally every 30 days:** If the frequency and duration result in reaching 30 calendar days from the previous therapy assessment prior to visit number 13 in a combined total, the reassessment is due prior to day 30. Counting is initiated on the first evaluation completed. There is no definition or time window for "minimally" so this can be scheduled for week two or three of care when anticipating reaching the 30-day requirement. Waiting until the last minute can create situations where reassessment visits are very close together or a patient cancellation risks compliance. When the first reassessment is completed, the 30-day calendar is reset, and the date of that visit is the starting point.

  – **Example 1:** The patient is receiving physical and occupational therapy with an expected plan that will cross 30 days before reaching a combined total of 13 visits. The occupational therapist completes her reassessment on visit 10 and the physical therapist completes his on visit 12.

  – **Example 2:** The patient began the episode with all three therapy services providing care and reached the 19th total visit during the first four weeks of care. The formal reassessment by physical therapy was completed on visit 16 and this resets the minimally every 30-day count specific to that discipline. As 30 calendar days from that reassessment approaches, only physical therapy remains active and schedules a reassessment visit on day 26. (Note: this day 26 is not day 26 of the certification episode but is day 26 in the specified 30-day count.)

♦ **13th total therapy visit:** When the combined total of therapy visits is going to reach 14 or more, a reassessment must be completed by any active therapy "close to" and possibly including the 13th visit. There is no defined range for "close to," so latitude is given based on patient situation.

  – **Example 3:** The patient is receiving all three therapy services with a planned total of 17 visits. Physical therapy completes the reassessment on visit 9, occupational therapy on visit 11, and speech-language pathology on visit 12.

- **Example 4:** The patient began services with occupational therapy and speech-language pathology. The combined total will be 15 visits. The occupational therapist completes her reassessment on visit 12. The speech-language pathologist completes a discharge assessment on visit 13.

- **19th total therapy visit:** When the combined total of therapy visits is going to reach 20 or more, a reassessment must be completed by any active therapy "close to" and possibly including the 19th visit. There is no defined range for "close to," so latitude is given based on patient situation.

  - **Example 5:** The patient is receiving all three therapy services with a planned total of 36 visits. In addition to the requirements of minimally 30 days and the 13th visit, physical therapy completes the reassessment on visit 18, occupational therapy on visit 16, and speech-language pathology on visit 17.

  - **Example 6:** The patient began services with occupational therapy and speech-language pathology. The combined total will be 25 visits. In addition to the requirements of minimally 30 days and the 13th visit, the occupational therapist completes her reassessment on visit 17. The speech-language pathologist completes a discharge assessment on visit 18.

- **Patient-driven exception:** Patient-specific situations may warrant the reassessment be completed earlier than the combined 13th or 19th visit and this is allowable.

There will be occasional situations in which the counting component will produce frustration and may lead to reassessments being close together. Visit data indicates that the majority of patients who receive 14 or more total therapy visits within an episode either start out as or have become single therapy cases, which should decrease the frequency of challenging scheduling issues.

Despite the logistical issues, periodic reevaluation of the care plan to confirm the effectiveness of therapy in home health is an important component of supporting medical necessity. It is an opportunity to put the pieces together and show the meaningful benefits to the patient as well as preserve the role of skilled therapy services in effective and efficient interdisciplinary care.

Therapy Requirements Fact Sheet

While changes to Publication 100-02, Chapter 7, Home Health Services are pending, the following information related to therapy requirements contained in the calendar year 2011 Final Home Health Rule is provided to assist home health aides and therapists with these requirements, effective April 1, 2011.

Assessment, measurement, and documentation of therapy effectiveness

To ensure therapy services are effective, at defined points during a course of treatment, for each therapy discipline for which services are provided, a qualified therapist (instead of an assistant) must perform the ordered therapy service. During this visit, the therapist must assess the patient using a method that allows for objective measurement of function and successive comparison of measurements. The therapist must document the measurement results in the clinical record. Specifically:

Initial therapy assessment

- For each therapy discipline for which services are provided, a qualified therapist (instead of an assistant) must assess the patient's function using a method that objectively measures activities of daily living such as, but not limited to, eating, swallowing, bathing, dressing, toileting, walking, climbing stairs, using assistive devices, and mental and cognitive factors. The measurement results must be documented in the clinical record.

- Where more than one discipline of therapy is being provided, a qualified therapist from each of the disciplines must functionally assess the patient. The therapist must document the measurement results, which correspond to the therapist's discipline and care plan goals, in the clinical record.

Reassessment at least every 30 days (performed in conjunction with an ordered therapy service)

- At least once every 30 days, for each therapy discipline for which services are provided, a qualified therapist (instead of an assistant) must provide the ordered therapy service, functionally reassess the patient, and compare the resultant measurement to prior assessment measurements. The therapist must document in the clinical record the measurement results along with the therapist's determination of the effectiveness of therapy, or lack thereof.

- Where more than one discipline of therapy is being provided, at least once every 30 days, a qualified therapist from each of the disciplines must provide the ordered therapy service, functionally reassess the patient, and compare the resultant measurement to prior assessment measurements. The therapist must document in the clinical record the measurement results along with the therapist's determination of the effectiveness of therapy, or lack thereof. In multidiscipline therapy cases, the qualified therapist would reassess functional items (and measure and document) those that correspond to the therapist's discipline and care plan goals.

Reassessment prior to the 14th and 20th therapy visit

- If a patient's course of therapy treatment reaches 13 therapy visits, for each therapy discipline for which services are provided, a qualified therapist (instead of an assistant) must provide the ordered 13th therapy service, functionally reassess the patient, and compare the resultant measurement to prior measurements. The therapist must document in the clinical record the measurement results along with the therapist's determination of the effectiveness of therapy, or lack thereof.

- Similarly, if a patient's course of therapy treatment reaches 19 therapy visits, a qualified therapist (instead of an assistant) must provide the ordered 19th therapy service and functionally reassess, measure, and document effectiveness of therapy, or lack thereof.

- When the patient resides in a rural area or when documented circumstances outside the control of the therapist prevent the qualified therapist's visit at exactly the 13th visit, the qualified therapist's visit can occur after the 10th therapy visit but no later than the 13th visit. Similarly, in rural areas or if documented exceptional circumstances exist, the qualified therapist's visit can occur after the 16th therapy visit but no later than the 19th therapy.

- Where more than one discipline of therapy is being provided, a qualified therapist from each of the disciplines must provide the ordered therapy service and functionally reassess, measure, and document the effectiveness of therapy or lack thereof close to but no later than the 13th and 19th therapy visit. The 13th and 19th therapy visit time points relate to the sum total of therapy visit from all therapy disciplines. In multidiscipline therapy cases, the qualified therapist would reassess functional items and measure those that correspond to the therapist's discipline and care plan goals.

- Therapy services provided after the 13th and 19th visit (sum total of therapy visit from all therapy disciplines) are not covered until:

  1. The qualified therapist(s) completes the assessment/measurement/documentation requirements.

  2. The qualified therapist(s) determines if the goals of the plan of care have been achieved or if the plan of care may require updating. If needed, changes to therapy goals or an updated plan of care is sent to the physician for signature or discharge.

  3. If the measurement results do not reveal progress toward therapy goals and/or do not indicate that therapy is effective, but therapy continues, the qualified therapist(s) must document why the physician and therapist have determined therapy should be continued.

Source: The Centers for Medicare & Medicaid Services. (2011). Therapy requirements fact sheet. Retrieved March 11, 2011, from www.cms.gov/HomeHealthPPS/Downloads/Therapy_Requirements_Fact_Sheet.pdf

Tips for Qualified Therapists

The amount of information and regulation that the home health therapist must understand and manage can be overwhelming. Documentation issues can seem secondary to clinical concerns but it is the delivery of efficient and effective care that ultimately creates documentation that clearly supports medical necessity. In an effort to promote improved focus and to move care forward, important elements of key issues as they relate to the qualified therapist have been compiled into a user-friendly format.

Outcome and Assessment Information Set (OASIS)

+ Completion of the OASIS tool is only one part of a comprehensive assessment at any time point: start of care, resumption of care, recertification, transfer, other follow-up, or discharge. Discipline- as well as agency-specific information must be included to create a detailed skilled visit.

+ The timing of the therapy assessment should allow the opportunity to provide collaborative information to improve the accuracy of OASIS data collection.

+ The intent of OASIS items that impact outcomes and risk adjustment should be considered as components of a thorough therapy assessment and meaningful care plan.

Assessments

+ Objective measurements are an integral component of supporting medical necessity. Although there are formal tools and tests available, it is important to recognize that measurements must be taken in a standardized manner.

+ Identified deficits, such as muscle weakness or limited range of motion, should be connected to a functional task to address "why" any difficulties are present. Assessments should include both the quantity and quality of performance.

+ Factors that can impact the course of care such as medication, visual, cognitive, or behavioral issues should be noted in the assessment.

Goals

+ Goal statements must be measurable and meaningful

+ Activities of daily living and instrumental activities of daily living goals should be task-specific and not treated as a group of activities

+ Goals must correlate to assessment findings and planned interventions

Planning Care

+ Interventions should be specific to issues identified during the assessment

+ "Training" is a category of activities and requires more detail to show why intervention is necessary

+ Orders should be as specific as possible and updated as needed

Routine Visits

+ Include what the therapist is contributing to impact the quality and quantity of patient performance; documentation should not read as repeated reassessments or observations of patient performance of activity

+ Be careful with documentation of therapeutic exercises—must be able to see what the therapist is doing beyond counting repetitions

+ "Teaching" risks appearing repetitive if there are insufficient details as to what is taught, any complicating factors, and how well the patient and/or caregiver is able to retain and implement information

Reassessments

+ Recertifications and reassessments must be completed by the physical therapist, occupational therapist, or speech-language pathologist; require an actual visit with the patient; and are considered a part of a treatment visit

+ Accurate timing requires active participation of the therapist in managing certification dates, calendar days, and visit counts

+ Reassessments focus on evaluating the effectiveness of therapy and making relevant changes to the plan of care based on clinical findings

Supervision of Assistants

+ Individual state requirements should be considered the minimum for regulatory compliance. The condition of the patient is a key factor in determining the level of involvement of the qualified therapist, which may need to be more frequent than dictated by the state practice act.

+ Supervision requires active communication and collaboration between the qualified therapist and the therapist assistant, and documentation should contain evidence of these specific activities.

+ Directing the plan of care is the responsibility of the qualified therapist. The decision to extend or discontinue any part or the entire plan is an ongoing activity throughout the episode that is based on objective assessments and clinical expertise. The presence of orders alone will not support medical necessity.

Tips for Therapist Assistants

As is true for the qualified therapist, the amount of information and regulation that the home health therapist assistant must understand and manage can be overwhelming. Documentation issues can seem secondary to clinical concerns, but it is the delivery of efficient and effective care that ultimately creates documentation that clearly supports medical necessity. In an effort to promote improved focus and to move care forward, important elements of key issues as they relate to therapist assistants have been compiled into a user-friendly format.

Outcome and Assessment Information Set (OASIS)

- Accuracy of OASIS data collection can be enhanced by collaboration and communication with therapist assistants, who need a basic working knowledge of the OASIS items

- Management of incontinence, interfering pain, and dyspnea are but a few examples of connecting the care provided by the therapist assistant to OASIS information

- A working knowledge of outcome measurements and process measures is necessary for therapist assistants to understand how the care delivered relates to these larger issues for home health

Assessments

- Information collected on the assessment must be communicated to the therapist assistant in a timely manner prior to the first visit he or she is going to complete. Verbal as well as written communication to direct the plan of care is required for safe patient care that follows the plan as designed.

- Although the formal assessment is not completed by the therapist assistant, feedback regarding the quality of the documentation provided in an assessment serves to enhance the ability to defend medical necessity.

- A level of assessment as to patient's progression toward goals, utilizing appropriate measures, is expected as part of the documentation provided by the therapist assistant.

Goals

- Goals should be considered on every visit to be clear about how the interventions planned for that particular patient encounter relate to them

- As patient progresses toward goals, communication with the qualified therapist to update as needed should occur on a regular basis and not just on the scheduled supervisory visits

- If it appears the goal is not attainable, timely communication with the qualified therapist is necessary to make any changes as indicated

Planning Care

- Feedback to the qualified therapist about the plan of care is an important component of elevating the quality of documentation and supporting medical necessity.

+ As the plan of care is moving forward, the need to add or remove interventions requires action by the qualified therapist after collaboration with the therapist assistant and shows clinical decision-making throughout the episode.

+ Addition of modalities to the plan of care requires a physician order and clear documentation that this was directed by the qualified therapist. This includes use of heating pads and ice packs the patient may already own.

Routine Visits

+ Include what the therapist assistant is contributing to impact the quality and quantity of patient performance; documentation should not read as repeated reassessments or observations of patient performance of activity

+ Be careful with documentation of therapeutic exercises—must be able to see what the therapist assistant is doing beyond counting repetitions

+ "Teaching" risks appearing repetitive if there are insufficient details as to what is taught, any complicating factors, and how well the patient and/or caregiver is able to retain and implement information

Reassessments

+ Accurate timing requires active participation of the therapist assistant in managing certification dates, calendar days, and visit counts

+ Feedback from the therapist assistant on the content of the documentation generated by a reassessment visit will provide an internal audit opportunity to confirm compliance

+ Changes to the plan of care as a result of the reassessment visit must be followed by the therapist assistant, and documentation should demonstrate consistency with those updates

Supervision of Assistants

- Individual state requirements should be considered the minimum for regulatory compliance. The condition of the patient is a key factor in determining the level of involvement of the qualified therapist, which may need to be more frequent than dictated by the state practice act.

- Supervision requires active two-way communication and collaboration between the qualified therapist and the therapist assistant, and documentation should contain evidence of these specific activities.

- Directing the plan of care is the responsibility of the qualified therapist. The decision to extend or discontinue any part or the entire plan is an ongoing activity throughout the episode that is based on objective assessments and clinical expertise. The presence of orders alone will not support medical necessity.

The Future of Therapy in Home Health

Documentation is clearly not a favorite topic of discussion for anyone in a medical profession. It can seem like just one more thing to add to the ever-growing pile of responsibilities on the shoulders of home health therapists. There is value in periodically climbing out of the tree to take a look at the forest and understand that concerns regarding the note generated on a single visit may appear as "no big deal" but that, in the larger picture, the role and impact of therapy in the home health setting is at stake. Decisions being made today regarding proposed care delivery models and payment restructuring that impact the industry as well as the continued move to reform the healthcare system will have far-reaching effects. It is important to look ahead and begin preparing for change now to secure the role of therapy as an integral part of the interdisciplinary team.

Payment for Home Health Services

The ultimate dissolution of the direct relationship between therapy visits and reimbursement in the Medicare Home Health Prospective Payment System is more a question of "when" than "if." After what appears to be a second consecutive shift in therapy visit numbers in response to a change in the payment structure, the concern regarding perceived incentives continues. The Medicare Payment Advisory Commission has recommended on several occasions that therapy utilization no longer be a factor in payment and a new model should be created that establishes reimbursement based on patient characteristics. Many therapists would welcome and embrace this type of patient-focused change. It will take time and resources for Medicare to develop and test a new model, and therapists are wise to want a seat at the table as this concept moves forward.

Medicare fee-for-service is not the only model of payment in home health. The impact of programs such as Medicare Advantage, health management organizations (HMO), Medicaid, as well as various private insurance companies has been felt by agencies to different degrees, depending on the area of the country they serve. Ongoing challenges to approval of necessary visits, criteria for coverage, and receiving payment that is adequate to cover costs are very real, and funds to pay for home health become increasingly limited.

As the industry waits to see how these plans unfold, the issue for all three therapies is to ensure that the value of therapy is clearly seen. The content of documentation supporting medical necessity and connecting to larger home health initiatives will be critical in defining the role of physical therapy, occupational therapy, and speech-language pathology in the provision of home health in the future.

Value-Based Purchasing

The tide is turning in healthcare from payment solely for the quantity of care—visits, procedures, days—to the additional element of the quality of care. The home health industry is essentially in the initial phases of this now as reimbursement is impacted by reporting Outcome and Assessment Information Set (OASIS) information to the Centers for Medicare & Medicaid Services (CMS). Agencies that do not submit OASIS data are subject to a reduction in payment. The next phase moves to payment based on measurable outcomes and, although this may be theoretical in some care settings, OASIS has collected more than 10 years of data about home health and outcome reporting, including Home Health Compare, that indicates we are well on our way.

Demonstration projects have been completed and therapists can stay informed using this link to the most current information: *hhp4p@cms.hhs.gov*. The future of therapy in home health will be defined by how well the focus and documentation of skilled care connects to outcomes as measured by OASIS. Therapists must begin to incorporate those concepts into their care planning and content now or risk being left behind as home health moves further down this road. What follows are a few highlights of some of the concepts and models that therapists should be aware of as healthcare reform unfolds.

Accountable Care Organizations

Although there are many details surrounding accountable care organizations (ACO) that require clarification as they become reality, the basic intent is similar to HMOs in that there is a shift in financial risk from the insurance company to the provider. The establishment of these ACOs will connect various healthcare settings, and home health agencies will need to position themselves as an integral part of any team. One of the themes is once again showing the value of care by managing costs effectively and achieving solid, measurable outcomes for the patients being served. The message of measurable quality is clear, and home health therapists need to be proactive in showing that their worth is more than revenue generation and be active participants in the development process in all care settings.

Medical Home Model

Using the definition provided by the Colorado Department of Public Health, the "Medical Home is not just a building, house or hospital, but a team approach to providing health care. A Medical Home originates in a primary health care setting that is family-centered and compassionate. A partnership develops between the family and the primary health care practitioner. Together they access all medical and non-medical services needed by the child and family to achieve maximum potential. The Medical Home maintains a centralized, comprehensive record of all health related services to promote continuity of care." It is clear that integrated care delivery across settings is one vision of healthcare reform that can impact therapy services in a variety of ways. Clearly demonstrating the medical necessity of the inclusion of physical therapy, occupational therapy, and speech-language pathology in any model will be met by the documentation being generated today—showing what is indispensable about every visit.

Continuity Assessment Record and Evaluation (CARE) Tool

As frustrated as therapists can be with OASIS, they may fall in love with it when learning that there is a new tool on the horizon. Some may long for a replacement of the current tool but be careful what is wished for. Considerable attention is being paid to the postacute continuum of care with respect to how, when, and why patients move between settings.

The Deficit Reduction Act of 2005 directed CMS to develop a postacute care payment reform demonstration. A report is due to be submitted to Congress in 2011. One component is the development of a standardized patient assessment tool used initially upon hospital discharge as well as when the patient is admitted to and discharged from a postacute setting. The CARE tool measures the clinical and functional status of Medicare patients at the time of acute discharge. It also measures changes in severity and other outcomes for patients receiving services in postacute settings.

Additional information can be found at *www.cms.gov*. The tool includes components that clearly indicate the influence of both the OASIS from home health and the minimum data set from skilled nursing facilities. The inclusion of the CARE tool in the discussion of therapy documentation is meant to reinforce that connecting what is traditionally seen as physical therapy, occupational therapy, and speech-language pathology to standardized tools such as OASIS will increase the ability to support the role of these services in care delivery as the industry continues to evolve.

Moving Forward

Coming full circle, the primary reason that high-quality therapists choose to practice in home health is the level of patient interaction and functionality unique to this setting. At the end of the day, the impact of even the smallest recommendation regarding mobility or self-care can be life-altering for patients and allow them to remain safely at home. Keeping the patient at the center of the discussion will keep the proper perspective on documentation. It is an extension and confirmation of the complexity of care that is going on every single day in homes across the country and validates physical therapy, occupational therapy, and speech-language pathology as key members of the interdisciplinary healthcare team now and in the future.

Overview of Home Health Quality Initiatives

In 2008, there were over 9,000 Medicare-certified home health agencies throughout the United States. In 2006, over 3 million beneficiaries were served and 103,931,188 visits made.

Home health is covered under the Part A Medicare benefit. It consists of part-time, medically necessary skilled care (nursing, physical therapy, occupational therapy, and speech-language therapy) that is ordered by a physician.

Quality healthcare for people with Medicare is a high priority for the Department of Health and Human Services, and CMS.

CMS has adopted the mission of the Institute of Medicine, who has defined quality as having the following properties or domains:

- Effectiveness: relates to providing care processes and achieving outcomes as supported by scientific evidence

- Efficiency: relates to maximizing the quality of a comparable unit of healthcare delivered or unit of health benefit achieved for a given unit of healthcare resources used

- Equity: relates to providing healthcare of equal quality to those who may differ in personal characteristics other than their clinical condition or preferences for care

- Patient centeredness: relates to meeting patients' needs and preferences and providing education and support

- Safety: relates to actual or potential bodily harm

- Timeliness: relates to obtaining needed care while minimizing delays

The instrument/data collection tool used to collect and report performance data by home health agencies is called OASIS. Since Fall 2003, CMS has posted on *www.medicare.gov* a subset of OASIS-based quality performance information showing how well home health agencies assist their patients in regaining or maintaining their ability to function.

Based on the 2005 National Quality Forum (NQF) endorsement, as of December 2007, 12 of these measures have been posted to Home Health Compare. The measures (all collected via the OASIS data set) are:

- Improvement in ambulation/locomotion

- Improvement in bathing

- Improvement in transferring

- Improvement in management of oral medication

- Improvement in pain interfering with activity

- Acute care hospitalization

- Emergent care

- Discharge to community

- Improvement in dyspnea (shortness of breath)

- Improvement in urinary incontinence

- Improvement in surgical wound status

- Emergent care for wound deterioration

At the request of CMS, NQF will review for potential endorsement a set of refined and newly developed home health measures in particular process measures for immunization, medication management, pain management, fall prevention, depression screening/intervention, care coordination, risk assessment, heart failure, and diabetes. These measures were tested in the revised OASIS tool.

NQF also will look to harmonize the home health measures with similar NQF-endorsed TM measures in other care settings (e.g., ambulatory, hospital, and nursing homes). NQF will work in partnership with the Agency for Healthcare Research and Quality and CMS, the accrediting entities, alliances, and representatives from major stakeholder groups to establish priorities and identify a set of national goals, measures corresponding to each goal, and a framework for accountability.

It is too early to know exactly how these changing priorities may impact the entire healthcare system. Planning/discussions are in a preliminary phase. Pay for performance logically will link to value and efficiency and actual activities and efforts of providers—using evidence-based practices and systems (in the form of process measures that will be collected at the agency level)—to promote use of such practices. Providers, consumers, and interested parties, such as the many organizations that represent and work with patients in postacute, home, community, and long-term care settings will be part of these efforts as they evolve. As we look to become stewards of the Medicare trusts funds, those that are quality- and mission-driven while maintaining some efficiencies will become increasingly important in transforming the healthcare system.

For more information on the Home Health Quality Initiatives, go to: *www.cms.gov/HomeHealthQualityInits*

Appendix

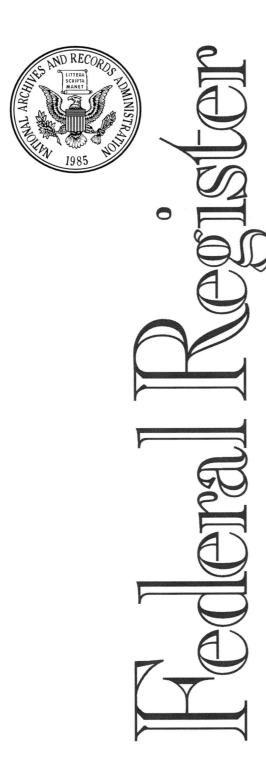

Wednesday,
November 17, 2010

Part II

Department of Health and Human Services

Center for Medicare & Medicaid Services

42 CFR Parts 409, 418, 424 et al.
Medicare Program; Home Health
Prospective Payment System Rate Update
for Calendar Year 2011; Changes in
Certification Requirements for Home
Health Agencies and Hospices; Final Rule

APPENDIX

DEPARTMENT OF HEALTH AND HUMAN SERVICES

Centers for Medicare & Medicaid Services

42 CFR Parts 409, 418, 424, 484, and 489

[CMS–1510–F]

RIN 0938–AP88

Medicare Program; Home Health Prospective Payment System Rate Update for Calendar Year 2011; Changes in Certification Requirements for Home Health Agencies and Hospices

AGENCY: Centers for Medicare & Medicaid Services (CMS), HHS.

ACTION: Final rule.

SUMMARY: This final rule sets forth an update to the Home Health Prospective Payment System (HH PPS) rates, including: the national standardized 60-day episode rates, the national per-visit rates, the nonroutine medical supply (NRS) conversion factors, and the low utilization payment amount (LUPA) add-on payment amounts, under the Medicare prospective payment system for HHAs effective January 1, 2011. This rule also updates the wage index used under the HH PPS and, in accordance with the Patient Protection and Affordable Care Act of 2010 (Affordable Care Act), updates the HH PPS outlier policy. In addition, this rule revises the home health agency (HHA) capitalization requirements. This rule further adds clarifying language to the "skilled services" section. The rule finalizes a 3.79 percent reduction to rates for CY 2011 to account for changes in case-mix, which are unrelated to real changes in patient acuity. Finally, this rule incorporates new legislative requirements regarding face-to-face encounters with providers related to home health and hospice care.

DATES: *Effective Date:* These regulations are effective on January 1, 2011.

FOR FURTHER INFORMATION CONTACT:

Frank Whelan, (410) 786–1302, for information related to payment safeguards.
Elizabeth Goldstein, (410) 786–6665, for CAHPS issues.
Mary Pratt, (410) 786–6867, for quality issues.
Randy Throndset, (410) 786–0131, for overall HH PPS issues.
Kathleen Walch, (410) 786–7970, for skilled services requirements and clinical issues.

Table of Contents

SUPPLEMENTARY INFORMATION:

I. Background

A. Statutory Background

The Balanced Budget Act of 1997 (BBA) (Pub. L. 105–33, enacted on August 5, 1997) significantly changed the way Medicare pays for Medicare home health (HH) services. Section 4603 of the BBA mandated the development of the home health prospective payment system (HH PPS). Until the implementation of an HH PPS on October 1, 2000, home health agencies (HHAs) received payment under a retrospective reimbursement system.

Section 4603(a) of the BBA mandated the development of an HH PPS for all Medicare-covered HH services provided under a plan of care (POC) that were paid on a reasonable cost basis by adding section 1895 of the Social Security Act (the Act), entitled "Prospective Payment For Home Health Services". Section 1895(b)(1) of the Act requires the Secretary to establish an HH PPS for all costs of HH services paid under Medicare.

Section 1895(b)(3)(A) of the Act requires the following: (1) The computation of a standard prospective payment amount includes all costs for HH services covered and paid for on a reasonable cost basis and that such amounts be initially based on the most recent audited cost report data available to the Secretary; and (2) the standardized prospective payment amount be adjusted to account for the effects of case-mix and wage level differences among HHAs.

Section 1895(b)(3)(B) of the Act addresses the annual update to the standard prospective payment amounts by the HH applicable percentage increase. Section 1895(b)(4) of the Act governs the payment computation. Sections 1895(b)(4)(A)(i) and (b)(4)(A)(ii) of the Act require the standard prospective payment amount to be adjusted for case-mix and geographic differences in wage levels. Section 1895(b)(4)(B) of the Act requires the establishment of an appropriate case-mix change adjustment factor for significant variation in costs among different units of services.

Similarly, section 1895(b)(4)(C) of the Act requires the establishment of wage adjustment factors that reflect the relative level of wages, and wage-related costs applicable to HH services furnished in a geographic area compared to the applicable national average level. Under section 1895(b)(4)(C) of the Act, the wage-adjustment factors used by the Secretary may be the factors used under section 1886(d)(3)(E) of the Act.

Section 1895(b)(5) of the Act, as amended by section 3131 of the Patient Protection and Affordable Care Act of 2010 (The Affordable Care Act) (Pub. L. 111–148, enacted on March 23, 2010) gives the Secretary the option to make additions or adjustments to the payment amount otherwise paid in the case of outliers because of unusual variations in the type or amount of medically necessary care. Section 3131(b) of the Affordable Care Act revised section 1895(b)(5) of the Act so that the standard payment amount is reduced by 5 percent and the total outlier payments in a given fiscal year (FY) or year may not exceed 2.5 percent of total payments projected or estimated. The provision also makes permanent a 10 percent agency level outlier payment cap.

In accordance with the statute, as amended by the BBA, we published a final rule in the July 3, 2000 **Federal Register** (65 FR 41128) to implement the

Finally, we would like to clarify that page 12 of the 2003 statement by the National Heart, Lung and Blood Institute (NHLBI) "Seventh Report of the Joint National Committee on Prevention, Detection, Evaluation, and Treatment of High Blood Pressure" (the JNC 7 report), published in the May 21, 2003, *Journal of the American Medical Association* explicitly states that prehypertension is not a disease category, which indicates that the coding of 401.1 or 401.9 for pre-hypertensive patients would not be appropriate. This is consistent with pre-existing ICD–9–CM guidance, which describes essential hypertension as SBP of 140 and above.

Comment: A commenter stated that the proposed 3.79 percent adjustment for nominal case-mix change appears to be based primarily on the inclusion of hypertension as a patient diagnosis and modified provision of therapy services consistent with the HH PPS model revision in 2008.

Response: As previously stated, the proposed adjustments for CY 2011 and CY 2012 took into account all of the nominal case-mix growth we measured between the IPS baseline and CY 2008, and netted out nominal case-mix growth that was already accounted for in previous rate reductions. As of last year's rate update regulation, we anticipated a need to compensate for a total nominal growth of 13.56 percent. This year's analysis showed that reductions previously planned to be implemented were not adequate to compensate for the full total of nominal growth (17.45 percent) that has occurred through 2008. Our method for deriving the real and nominal case-mix change percentages did not isolate any specific sources of nominal growth (such as hypertension coding) upon which to base the reduction. However, the proposed rule for CY 2011 described statistics showing a large 1-year increase in hypertension reporting between 2007 and 2008, and it noted that the observed growth in the numbers of episodes with high numbers of therapy visits was unexpected. The proposed rule also discussed evidence beyond hypertension and therapy, such as increased reporting of secondary diagnoses in general.

In summary, in this final rule, we are implementing the proposed 3.79 percent reduction to the national standardized episode rate for CY 2011. We will defer finalizing a payment reduction for CY 2012 until further study of the case-mix change data and/or methodology is completed. In addition, in this rule, we are withdrawing the proposal to apply the case-mix change reduction to the NRS conversion factor. As part of our

review of the nominal case-mix change methodology, we will study its applicability to the NRS model. The NRS conversion factor will be updated in CY 2011 by the market basket update of 1.1 percent and will also be adjusted for outlier payments in accordance with section 3131(b) of the Affordable Care Act. We are also withdrawing our proposal to eliminate ICD9–CM diagnosis codes 401.1, Benign Essential Hypertension, and 401.9, Unspecified Essential Hypertension, from the HH PPS case-mix model's hypertension group, pending the results of a more comprehensive analysis of the resource use of patients with these conditions.

B. Therapy Clarifications

In the CY 2011 HH PPS proposed rule, we discussed analyses that suggested that therapy under the Medicare HH benefit, in many cases, was being over-utilized. Analysis of HH utilization under the original single 10-visit therapy threshold suggests that the threshold offered a strong financial incentive to provide therapy visits when a lower amount of therapy was more clinically appropriate. Essentially, the data suggested that financial incentives to provide 10 therapy visits overpowered clinical considerations in therapy prescriptions. For the CY 2008 final rule, we established a system of three thresholds (6, 14, and 20 therapy visits) with graduated steps in between to meet our objectives of retaining the prospective nature of the payment system, reducing the strong incentive resulting from the single 10 therapy threshold, restoring clinical considerations in therapy provision, and paying more accurately for therapy utilization below the 10-visit therapy threshold.

In the proposed rule, we described that analysis of CY 2008 data continues to suggest that some HHAs may be providing unnecessary therapy. MedPAC states in its March 2010 report that 2008 data also reveal a 26 percent increase of episodes with 14 or more therapy visits (MedPAC, *Report to Congress: Medicare Payment Policy*, Section B, Chapter 3, March 2010, p. 203). While this analysis suggested that therapy payment policies are vulnerable to fraud and abuse, the swift, across-the-board therapy utilization changes also suggest another more fundamental concern. MedPAC wrote in the March 2010 report (MedPAC, 2010, p. 206) that payment incentives continue to influence treatment patterns, and that payment policy is such a significant factor in treatment patterns because the criteria for receipt of the HH benefit are ill-defined. MedPAC also reported that

better guidelines would facilitate more appropriate use of the benefit.

As such, in the CY 2011 HH PPS proposed rule, we proposed to clarify our policies regarding coverage of therapy services at § 409.44(c) in order to assist HHAs and to curb misuse of the benefit. Specifically, we proposed the following:

• Require that measurable treatment goals be described in the plan of care and that the patient's clinical record would demonstrate that the method used to assess a patient's function would include objective measurement and successive comparison of measurements, thus enabling objective measurement of progress toward goals and/or therapy effectiveness.

• Require that a qualified therapist (instead of an assistant) perform the needed therapy service, assess the patient, measure progress, and document progress toward goals at least once least every 30 days during a therapy patient's course of treatment. For those patients needing 13 or 19 therapy visits, we proposed to require that a qualified therapist (instead of an assistant) perform the therapy service required at the 13th or 19th visit, assess the patient, and measure and document effectiveness of the therapy. We would cease coverage of therapy services if progress towards plan of care goals cannot be measured, unless the documentation supports the expectation that progress can be expected in a reasonable and predictable timeframe. An exception to this would be when the criteria for needing maintenance therapy are met.

• Clarify when the establishment and performance of a maintenance program is covered therapy.

Comment: A number of commenters were in strong support of our efforts to rein in abuse and overuse of therapy through sound documentation, objective measurement, and appropriate involvement of qualified therapists. Commenters expressed support for proposed additional requirements of documentation of the patient's clinical record, including therapy treatment goals to be described in the plan of care and objective measurement obtained during the functional assessment. One commenter stated that the elements of documentation added in our proposed regulations are reflective of professional standards for the practice of speech-language pathology. Another commenter expressed general support of our therapy coverage and documentation requirements, including those for patient assessment, physician collaboration, plan of care, goal establishment, evaluation of progress

70390 Federal Register / Vol. 75, No. 221 / Wednesday, November 17, 2010 / Rules and Regulations

toward goals through objective measures, and documentation, indicating they are all reflective of professional standards of practice for therapy services, such as those established by named major therapy associations. Another commenter expressed support for the proposed therapy coverage requirements regarding functional assessments, treatment plan revisions, and accurate documentation, indicating that these requirements align with professional standards of clinical practice.

Response: We thank the commenters for their support.

Comment: Numerous commenters expressed concern regarding the provision of the proposed rule requiring that a qualified therapist, instead of an assistant, perform the needed therapy service at the 13th and 19th therapy visits. These commenters stated that therapy visits by a qualified therapist beyond those already conducted on the 1st, 30th, and 60th days would be prohibitively expensive to HHAs and an unnecessary intrusion for patients. A number of commenters suggested that requiring a qualified therapist, instead of an assistant, to perform the needed therapy service every 30 days should be sufficient, stating that requiring a qualified therapist to perform the therapy service on the 13th and 19th visits was excessive. A commenter suggested that because only 15 percent of episodes contained more than 13 therapy visits and only 5 percent of episodes contained more than 19 therapy visits, CMS should consider the increased costs of its proposed required therapy changes versus the actual need for the new requirement. Commenters quoted recent findings of a health care consulting company's survey of HH providers regarding the proposed therapy clarifications, stating that most providers believe the proposed therapy changes would lead to scheduling difficulties for therapy visits and would cause difficulties in employing/contracting qualified therapists. A few commenters asked CMS to delay the implementation date of this provision by one quarter to allow more transition time for providers. Several commenters suggested, as an alternative to the requirement that a qualified therapist perform the needed therapy service at the 13th and 19th visit, that adopting ranges would be more acceptable—for example, allowing the qualified therapist visit to occur between the 11th and 13th visits and again between the 17th and 19th visits. Another commenter proposed that CMS should instead defer to State law requirements, asserting that most States require more

frequent qualified therapist supervision of assistants than those in the proposed rule, and the proposal's timeframes would be redundant to State laws. The commenter further stated that the proposed defined timeframes are in conflict with § 409.44(a) as they fail to reflect attention to the patient's individual needs. Further, the commenter suggested that CMS abandon the 13th and 19th qualified therapist visit requirement and instead base the reassessment timeframe on individual care needs and changes in patient status. That same commenter added that assistants utilize their clinical reasoning skills every time they treat a patient and advise the supervising therapist regarding the patient's need for continued skill intervention and grading of treatment and, therefore, the requirement for qualified therapist visits at defined timeframes is not reasonable. A commenter classified all our proposed therapy visit rules as arbitrary at best, as well as calling these latest rules regarding the 13th and 19th assessments capricious. One commenter stated that a requirement to re-evaluate patients at the 13th and 19th visits may not be effective in curbing agencies from inappropriately using the benefit in the long-run, suggesting that some agencies will soon learn how to work the revised system to their benefit. A commenter stated that, while overall therapy utilization has increased, it has led to better outcomes for Medicare beneficiaries and overall spending per Medicare patient has remained well below Congressional Budget Office (CBO) projections. Referring to the aforementioned survey results, the commenter described the surveyed HHAs' concern that the proposed clarifications would result in limited improvements in patient care. Several commenters believed that the proposed changes would have an adverse effect on access to care and timeliness of services provided and that these requirements would result in less direct patient care time. Many commenters stated that the documentation requirements were burdensome and costly. Several commenters feared that these requirements would impede access to care in rural areas where there are shortages of qualified therapists.

Response: We thank the commenters for their suggestions. We continue to believe that to ensure Medicare HH patients receive effective, high-quality therapy services, the frequency that a qualified therapist must assess the effectiveness of services performed by assistants must be more clearly defined in Medicare home health coverage

regulations. Longstanding Medicare Conditions of Participation (CoPs) regulations at § 484.32(a) require that HH therapy services be administered by a qualified therapist or a qualified assistant under the therapist's supervision, thus requiring a qualified therapist to supervise therapy services to ensure their effectiveness. We believe that in order to adhere to these regulations, a qualified therapist must periodically perform the patient's needed therapy service during the course of treatment to ensure that the therapy being provided by assistants is effective and/or that the patient is progressing toward treatment goals. These visits ensure that the qualified therapist has first-hand knowledge of the patient in order to identify needed changes to the care plan. Additionally, these visits enable a qualified therapist to determine if treatment goals have been achieved or if therapy has ceased to be effective. We note that some States preclude assistants by scope of practice from making determinations such as whether goals are met. As such, we believe that by requiring a qualified therapist, instead of an assistant, to perform the needed therapy service, assess the patient, and measure and document progress toward goals and/or effectiveness of therapy at defined points in the course of treatment, we would lessen the risk that patients continue to receive therapy after the treatment goals have been reached and/or after therapy is no longer effective.

In response to the commenter who stated that while overall therapy utilization has increased, such increased utilization has led to better outcomes for Medicare beneficiaries, we disagree with the conclusion. In their March 2010 report, MedPAC described that functional measure scores for HH patients continue to improve, but also expressed concerns that the measures may not appropriately depict the quality of therapy provided by HHAs. MedPAC reports that there are no measures, which reflect functional improvement for only those patients that receive therapy services. Instead, the measures reflect functional improvement for all patients. Therefore, we believe that the data do not support the commenter's conclusion that higher volumes of therapy have led to better outcomes. The same commenter, pointing to results of the survey described above, stated that the HHAs believe these proposed therapy coverage clarifications would result in limited improvements in patient care. Again, we disagree with these opinions. We refer the commenter to research studies conducted by Linda

Federal Register / Vol. 75, No. 221 / Wednesday, November 17, 2010 / Rules and Regulations   **70391**

Resnick (of Brown University) et al., entitled "Predictors of Physical Therapy Clinic Performance in the Treatment of Patients with Low Back Pain Syndromes" (2008, funded by a grant from the National Institute of Child Health) and "State Regulation and the Delivery of Physical Therapy Services" (2006, funded in part through a grant from the Agency for Healthcare Research and Quality). Both studies concluded that more therapy time spent with a qualified physical therapist, and less time with a physical therapist assistant, is more efficient and leads to better patient outcomes. In these studies, the lower percentage of time seen by a qualified therapist and the greater percentage of time seen by an assistant or aide, the more likely a patient would have more visits per treatment per episode. The studies also concluded that, although delegation of care to therapy support personnel such as assistants may extend the productivity of the qualified physical therapist, it appears to result in less efficient and effective services. We believe that by requiring regular visits by a qualified therapist during a course of treatment we will achieve more appropriate and efficient provision of therapy services while also achieving better therapy outcomes. Regarding the comment that HH expenditures are below CBO projections, we are unclear on the commenter's suggestion. We believe that the commenter may have been suggesting that the growth in HH expenditures does not warrant our attempts to facilitate more appropriate and effective therapy utilization. If so, we disagree with the commenter. We continue to believe that these improved guidelines, as suggested by MedPAC, are an important step in addressing program vulnerabilities while also improving the quality of services provided. We also disagree with the commenters who believe that a qualified therapist visit every 30 days is sufficient, and that the required 13th and 19th visits are excessive and redundant to many state practice supervision requirements, and that the 13th and 19th visit requirement timeframes fail to reflect the patient's individual needs. As we have noted in this and previous rules, at the inception of the HH PPS we analyzed the amount of therapy a HH rehabilitation patient would typically require during a course of treatment. We used clinical judgment to determine that the typical rehabilitation patient in a HH setting would require about 8 hours of therapy, or 10 therapy visits during a course of treatment. We believe that when the

unique condition of an individual patient requires more therapy than a typical Medicare HH rehabilitation patient, such a patient should be more closely monitored by a qualified therapist to ensure that high-quality, effective services are being provided and/or acceptable progress toward goals is being achieved. We also continue to believe that to ensure that this monitoring occurs for all high-therapy needs Medicare patients, we cannot depend on individual state supervision requirements. Instead, Medicare coverage clarifications will ensure that all Medicare HH patients benefit from this oversight. We also disagree with commenters that these policies will lead to an intrusion for patients. To the contrary, research suggests that more qualified therapist involvement would further enhance patient care for those patients needing these levels of therapy. We also note that these policies will not result in additional visits or therapy services provided to the patient. The visit by a qualified therapist would not be in addition to the visit that would otherwise occur, as described in the patient's treatment plan. Instead, the qualified therapist, perhaps instead of an assistant, would perform the therapy service at defined points in the course of treatment. In response to the commenter who questioned whether a comprehensive assessment of the patient would need to occur during these qualified therapist visits, we refer the commenter to the regulation text changes at § 409.44(c)(1)(iv) which describes that the qualified therapist must assess a patient's function using objective measurement of function. In other words, the assessment of function would not be a comprehensive assessment of the patient's clinical condition.

In response to the commenters who expressed cost and access to care concerns associated with these policies we note that current CoPs at § 484.12 already require that the HHA and its staff comply with accepted professional standards and principles that apply to professionals furnishing services by a HHA. Those accepted professional standards include complete and effective documentation, such as that which we described in our proposal. (Section 484.55 of the CoPs already requires that HHAs provide a comprehensive assessment that "accurately reflects the patient's current health status and includes information that may be used to demonstrate progress toward achievement of desired outcomes.") In addition, § 484.2 requires that a clinical note be a notation of

contact with a patient that is written and dated by a member of the health team, and that describes signs and symptoms, treatment and drugs administered and the patient's reaction, and any changes in physical or emotional condition, which becomes part of the medical record. Further, § 484.48, our longstanding regulation for CoPs and clinical records, requires that a clinical record containing pertinent past and current findings in accordance with accepted professional standards be maintained for every patient receiving HH services. In addition to the plan of care, the record must include treatment plans and activity orders, signed, and dated clinical and progress notes, and copies of summary reports sent to the attending physician. Because these proposed clarifications to our therapy coverage requirements are consistent with long-standing CoP requirements and accepted professional standards of clinical practice, we would expect that many providers have already adopted these practices.

Also, because CoPs at § 484.32 allow therapy services offered by the HHA to be provided by a qualified therapist or a qualified assistant under the supervision of qualified therapist and in accordance with the plan of care, it is our expectation that HHAs are already utilizing qualified therapists regularly to perform the needed therapy services in order to perform the required supervision of assistants.

We agree with the commenter that most HH therapy patients do not receive 13 and/or 19 visits in their course of treatment. In response to the comments which stated the relatively small numbers do not warrant the 13 and 19 qualified therapist visit and documentation requirements, suggesting instead that we target providers with suspect therapy practices for review, we reiterate that we believe these requirements benefit all patients. We believe that these requirements may also deter inappropriate provision of high levels of therapy, and therefore lessen the risk of the associated inappropriate higher HH PPS payments. In summary, by requiring qualified therapist visits when the amount of therapy reaches those high levels, which also correspond to high payment levels, we believe we can simultaneously achieve better patient outcomes, more efficient provision of therapy, and more accurate reimbursement.

We find compelling the commenters' concerns regarding scheduling difficulties. We believe the commenters' concerns regarding scheduling warrant more flexibility in the timing of the 13th and 19th visit requirements. Therefore,

70392 **Federal Register** / Vol. 75, No. 221 / Wednesday, November 17, 2010 / Rules and Regulations

we have decided to allow for some flexibility associated with the 13th and 19th therapy visit rule for patients. Specifically, for beneficiaries in rural areas, the qualified therapist may perform the needed therapy service, reassessment and measurement at any time after the 10th therapy visit but no later than the 13th therapy visit, and after the 16th therapy visit but no later than the 19th therapy visit. And, if extenuating circumstances outside the control of the therapist preclude the therapy service visit, reassessment and measurement at the 13th and 19th timeframes, the qualified therapist may perform the therapy service visit, reassessment and measurement at any time after the 10th therapy visit but no later than the 13th therapy visit, and after the 16th therapy visit but no later than the 19th therapy visit.

Regarding the access to care concerns, we believe that these requirements will ultimately result in more access to effective therapy services. MedPAC reports broad access to HH care for Medicare beneficiaries. As such, we do not expect that these coverage clarifications will result in access to care issues, but we will monitor for unanticipated effects.

We note, however, because of the volume of comments we received on this issue, we believe that many agencies have not been in compliance with the documentation practices and qualified therapist oversight we would expect. Therefore, we have decided to delay the effective date of these requirements until April 1, 2011, to allow agencies that do not currently have such practices in place additional time to transition.

Comment: A number of commenters expressed support for our efforts to require reassessments, but had questions as to how assessment visit requirements at the 13th and 19th visit would work when multiple therapy disciplines are providing care. Specifically, commenters stated that because HH therapy can consist of any combination of three therapy disciplines, it would be difficult for therapists to track the 13th and 19th visits if more than one therapy discipline was serving the patient. Commenters asked how it would be determined which therapist would do the 13th and 19th assessments. Additionally, commenters were concerned that CMS might be expecting a therapist of one discipline to do the assessment for the therapist of another discipline. Commenters stated that it would be unrealistic and cumbersome to track the 13th and 19th visits, especially when there are multiple

therapy disciplines involved. In a related comment, a commenter recommended further clarification of the proposed regulations by requesting that CMS further specify that professional standards should be those pertaining to the individual professions. The commenter also stated that, because existing Medicare regulations require compliance with Federal, State, and local laws, requiring the proposed qualified therapist visits at defined points in the course of treatment could contradict State licensure and scope of practice laws.

Response: We concur with the commenters that we need to clarify our expectation when more than one therapy discipline is providing services to the patient. We will clarify the regulation text to state that the policy applies to each discipline separately. The patient's function must be initially assessed and periodically reassessed by a qualified therapist of the corresponding discipline for the type of therapy being provided (that is, PT, OT, and/or SLP). When more than one therapy discipline is being provided, the corresponding qualified therapist would perform the reassessment during the regularly scheduled visit associated with that discipline which was scheduled to occur as near as possible to the 13th and 19th visit, but no later than the 13th and 19th visit.

We also note that a small percentage of patients which receive 13 and 19 therapy visits receive more than 1 therapy discipline. In addition, HHAs must coordinate their patients' care per longstanding conditions of participation at § 484.14(g). As such, we would expect such coordination to already be occurring. Given the low volume of such patients and the added flexibility as described above, we do not believe that the coordination associated with multi-therapy discipline patients will be overly burdensome. However, we will monitor the effects of this provision to identify unintended consequences.

Comment: Several commenters suggested that instead of putting additional requirements on all HHAs in response to a smaller number of HHAs who are abusing the system, CMS should target those agencies that are providing unnecessary therapy. A few commenters urged CMS to consider how the therapy provisions of this rule would affect HHAs, especially in rural areas, where there is a shortage of therapists. A commenter also stated that the notion that HH expenditures were high due to unnecessary therapy visits is inaccurate and provided statistics that he believes prove therapy overutilization is not a problem.

Response: As we have described in previous comment responses, we believe that these proposed requirements will strengthen the integrity of the benefit while also resulting in better patient outcomes. We believe all HHAs, not just suspect agencies, should adhere to these best practices in order to provide high-quality and effective therapy services, consistent with existing CoPs.

Comment: A few commenters expressed concern regarding therapy services possibly not being covered after a hospitalization, as a result of these assessment visit requirements. Specifically, the commenters were concerned that we were imposing new limits on maintenance therapy. Commenters expressed fear that the result of not covering such therapy services might be that many high fall risk patients would be sent home without therapy care, which would lead to increased falls/hospitalizations/ fractures that would increase Medicare spending in the end. Another commenter stated that physical therapy and occupational therapy were utilized more for safety evaluations and fall prevention measures, especially for patients on medication, which places them at a higher risk for falls. This commenter added that fall prevention best practice interventions provided in patients' homes save Medicare money. Similarly, a commenter asked CMS to clarify therapy coverage for pain.

Response: We agree with the commenter that fall prevention practices and/or pain management are essential for many HH patients in order to provide the patient with quality care. We remind the commenter that a longstanding coverage requirement for HH therapy services under Medicare is that the services which the patient needs must require the performance by or supervision of a qualified therapist. Whether or not fall prevention services and pain management services are covered therapy depends on the unique clinical condition of the patient and the complexity of the needed therapy services. Many fall prevention services would not require the skills of a therapist. Longstanding regulations allow therapy coverage when, for safety and effectiveness reasons, the unique medical complexities of the patient require a qualified therapist's skills in the establishment or performance of a therapy maintenance program. As such, should the unique clinical condition of a patient require that the specialized skills, knowledge, and judgment of a qualified therapist are needed to design and establish a safe and effective maintenance program in connection with a specific illness or injury, then such services would be covered as therapy services.

Comment: Commenters were opposed to the requirement that a skilled nursing service must be needed in order to have maintenance therapy covered, and that a maintenance program cannot be established after restorative therapy has ended.

Response: The intent of language in the proposed rule was to clarify that, in order for the establishment of a maintenance therapy program to be considered covered therapy, the specialized skills, knowledge, and judgment of a therapist would be required in developing a maintenance program. Services would be covered to design or establish the plan, to ensure patient safety, to train the patient, family members and/or unskilled personnel in carrying out the maintenance plan, and to make periodic reevaluations of the plan. In the proposed rule, we further noted scenarios in which maintenance therapy may be provided in the home setting.

The language in the proposed rule was not meant to indicate that maintenance therapy could not be provided as the sole skilled service and would be covered only if ancillary to another skilled qualifying service. The proposed clarifications were not intended to expand or limit existing coverage criteria. We regret the confusion these scenarios may have caused. We note that therapy coverage criteria have always been based on the inherent complexity of the service which the patient needs. As such, maintenance therapy has and will continue to be covered in the HH setting when the unique clinical condition of the patient requires the complex services which can only be provided effectively and safely by a qualified therapist. We will revise the proposed regulation text to address the commenters' confusion.

Comment: A number of commenters expressed concern regarding proposed regulation text changes that state therapy visits would not be covered for transient or easily reversible loss or reduction in function. Some commenters who opposed the proposed regulation text changes stated that these changes would disallow coverage of maintenance therapy, citing longstanding Medicare HH coverage policies previously set out in the "Health Insurance For the Aged, Home Health Agency Manual," Pub. 11 (HIM–11) that allowed for the coverage of such maintenance therapy. One commenter recommended striking the language, "transient and reversible loss." A

commenter also stated that these proposed regulation changes are in direct conflict with section 1814(a)(2)(C) of the Act. Commenters questioned what criteria define a transient and reversible reduction in function, or when a patient's condition could be expected to improve spontaneously. One commenter stated that it is difficult to determine when conditions are or are not transient and reversible, noting that some patients who present a very serious condition on admission may recover quickly, while others with seemingly less-serious conditions can end up being far more complex as treatments progress. Another commenter stated we must take into account the patient's unique condition.

Response: We disagree with the commenter that the proposed regulation text changes conflict with section 1814(a)(2)(C) of the Act. We believe that the commenter is inferring that by not allowing therapy coverage for an easily reversible reduction in function, we would be denying coverage to a patient who needs therapy, an eligibility criterion listed in section 1814(a)(2)(C) of the Act. We disagree with such interpretation. Consistent with statute, longstanding regulation, and longstanding manual guidance, therapy coverage under the HH benefit is based on a patient's need for skilled services. The therapy services must be of such a level of complexity and sophistication or the condition of the beneficiary must be such that the services required can safely and effectively be performed only by a qualified therapist or a qualified therapy assistant under the supervision of a qualified therapist. Services which do not require the performance or supervision of a qualified therapist are not reasonable and necessary services, even if they are performed by a qualified therapist.

When a patient suffers a transient and easily reversible loss or reduction of function which could reasonably be expected to improve spontaneously as the patient gradually resumes normal activities, the services do not require the performance or supervision of a qualified therapist, and those services are not considered reasonable and necessary covered therapy services. We acknowledge that making a determination that a patient suffers a transient and easily reversible loss or reduction of function which could reasonably be expected to improve spontaneously as the patient gradually resumes normal activities requires clinical judgment and a consideration of the patient's unique condition. We believe that rehabilitation professionals, by virtue of their education and

experience, are typically able to determine when a functional impairment could reasonably be expected to improve spontaneously as the patient gradually resumes normal activities. Likewise, we expect rehabilitation professionals to be able to recognize when their skills are appropriate to promote recovery. A prescriptive definition of these sorts of conditions, such as a listing of specific disease states that provide subtext for these descriptions is impractical, as each patient's recovery from illness is based on unique characteristics. In response to the commenter who believes that the therapy clarifications would disallow coverage of maintenance therapy, we assure the commenter that these clarifications do not impose new limits on the criteria for maintenance therapy coverage. We again note that therapy coverage criteria have always been based on the inherent complexity of the service which the patient needs. As such, maintenance therapy has and will continue to be covered in the HH setting when the unique clinical condition of the patient requires the complex services, which can only be provided effectively and safely by a qualified therapist. In addition, we note that these clarifications are consistent with longstanding manual guidance.

Comment: A commenter urged CMS to address therapy coverage for conditions that may not directly impact functional status, such as the role of therapists in wound care.

Response: We reiterate that if the services do not require the performance or supervision of a qualified therapist, those services are not considered to be reasonable and necessary covered therapy services. As such, if a therapist (who is qualified to do so per her or his State Practice Act) would perform services such as wound-care, those services would be covered therapy only if they required the skills of the qualified therapist or qualified assistant under the supervision of a qualified therapist. Should a qualified therapist (who is qualified to do so per her or his State Practice Act) perform wound care that does not require the specialized skills of a therapist and could be routinely performed by agency nursing staff, these services would not be covered therapy services.

Comment: A commenter expressed concern over the proposed therapy coverage clarifications, stating that the proposed regulatory text changes are major changes to current policy and that they are in conflict with Medicare statute and current law. The commenter stated that Medicare coverage will be more difficult to obtain for beneficiaries with chronic and debilitating conditions if the proposals are finalized. The commenter urged CMS to withdraw the maintenance therapy regulation text changes, stating that maintenance therapy is a covered benefit in home health and that Medicare statute does not require improvement for services to qualify for coverage. The commenter stated that the restoration potential of a patient is not the deciding factor in determining whether skilled services are needed, further stating that even if full recovery or medical improvement is not possible, a patient may need skilled services to prevent further deterioration or preserve current capabilities. The commenter stated that a prescribed therapy service which requires the skills of a therapist to help maintain function or prevent slow deterioration is medically necessary and should be covered under the statute. The commenter stated that current regulations recognize this, but the proposed changes minimize this point, and the commenter urged CMS to not restrict benefits in order to fight fraud.

The commenter expressed concern with the proposal's use of the words "improvement" and "progress," fearing an increased emphasis on these terms in the rules for therapy coverage will limit access to care for patients who require maintenance therapy. Further, the commenter alleged that the proposed rule would require improvement for therapy to be covered. The commenter suggested the word "effective" is more appropriate than "improvement" or "progress."

The commenter believed that the proposed regulation text will require the therapist to use complex and sophisticated therapy techniques in order for maintenance therapy to be covered and will thus be a new coverage limitation preventing needed access to therapy, and that the proposed regulation text which states that maintenance therapy must be required in connection with a specific disease would also newly limit maintenance therapy coverage. Further, the commenter alleged that the revised regulation text does not consider the unique condition of the patient as it must and as does the current regulation text. The commenter stated that the proposal newly categorizes maintenance therapy as not rehabilitative, while the current regulations include both restorative and maintenance therapy as rehabilitative. The commenter stated that, should CMS require improvement as a therapy coverage criterion, CMS would be applying an arbitrary "rule of thumb" which does not consider the patient's individual condition, and such

a requirement for improvement conflicts with the current regulation at § 409.42. Further, the commenter stated that the proposed regulation text changes will result in denials of Medicare coverage for beneficiaries with long-term, progressive, or incurable conditions. The commenter also took issue with the proposed regulation text change to require the documentation of progress toward goals.

The commenter further stated that the definition of maintenance therapy is too vague and restrictive. The commenter also took issue with the proposed regulation text, which requires that, in order for maintenance therapy to be covered, the skills of a therapist must be needed to ensure the patient's safety "and" the skills of a therapist are needed to provide a safe and effective maintenance program. The commenter believed that we should replace the "and" with an "or". The commenter also stated that the regulation does not define "reasonable and necessary" in a way that clearly provides for coverage of maintenance therapy. As was also mentioned by other commenters, this commenter was concerned that the proposed regulation text describes coverage of the development of a maintenance program during the last visit(s) for rehabilitative therapy, stating that, often, standard practice is to establish and instruct the patient in an appropriate maintenance program at the outset of a course of therapy. The commenter also spoke to the proposed regulation text change, which appears to indicate that we would not cover the establishment of a maintenance program after a restorative therapy program has ended, or if a beneficiary had never met the criteria for restorative therapy. The commenter stated that the proposed regulation text would result in maintenance therapy becoming a dependent service.

Response: The proposed regulatory text clarifications are intended to neither limit nor expand the coverage of therapy in the HH setting, but instead are intended to provide clear therapy guidelines, as suggested by MedPAC, to deter inappropriate provisions of therapy services. As we have described in earlier responses to comments, we also believe that these guidelines will improve patient outcomes, improve therapy effectiveness, and promote more consistent compliance with the Medicare CoPs. However, as we described in an earlier comment response, we agree with the commenter that the proposed regulation text changes may have been unclear in the descriptive scenarios surrounding coverage of the development of a

maintenance program, and we will revise the final regulation text changes at § 409.44(c)(2)(iii)(B) to remove the scenarios described in the proposed rule's § 409.44(c)(2)(iii)(B)(1) through (B)(3).

We also agree with the commenter that there are some additional changes to the proposed regulation text that we should finalize for better clarity. We believe that these changes may alleviate some of the commenter's concerns that the proposed rule limits coverage associated with maintenance therapy, and reassure the commenter that the coverage criteria clarifications are consistent with statute, current regulations, and longstanding manual guidance. Specifically, in response to the commenter's concern that we would have newly categorized maintenance therapy as non-rehabilitation, we will delete the proposed regulation text at § 409.44(c)(2)(iii)(A)(2) and (A)(3) for the final rule. We believe our attempts to clarify these definitions are not needed, as those definitions are well defined in § 409.44(c)(2)(iii)(A) through (iii)(C). We will also finalize some technical changes to the proposed regulation text, including replacing several of the proposed regulatory text references to improvements in function with references to the effectiveness of the care plan goals, as suggested by the commenter.

We agree with the commenter that current regulations and longstanding manual guidance are consistent in that therapy services are covered in the HH setting based on the inherent complexity of the service which the patient needs. As such, maintenance therapy has and will continue to be covered in the HH setting when the unique clinical condition of the patient requires the complex services, which can only be provided effectively and safely by a qualified therapist.

Regarding the commenter's concern that the proposed rule stated that skilled therapy is not reasonable and necessary unless improvement is documented, we disagree with the commenter's interpretation of the proposed rule. However, we agree that we could have been more clear in the regulation text which describes the documentation requirements at § 409.44(c)(2)(i). In the final rule, we will clearly state that maintenance therapy as defined in § 409.44(c)(2)(iii)(B) and § 409.44(c)(2)(iii)(C) would not be subject to the criteria listed in § 409.44(c)(2)(i)(B)(4).

Concerning the comment that the proposed regulation text, which requires the therapist to use complex and sophisticated therapy techniques in order for maintenance therapy to be covered, imposes a new coverage limitation associated with maintenance therapy and will prevent needed access to therapy, we refer the commenter to longstanding manual guidance at 40.2.2 E. in chapter 7 of the Medicare Benefit Policy Manual, CMS Pub. 100–2. This section contains longstanding guidance which uses the term "complex and sophisticated procedures" when describing reasonable and necessary maintenance therapy. This same chapter instructs a reviewer to consider the inherent complexity of the service when determining if the skills of a therapist are required. The complexity and sophistication of the service are longstanding criteria used to assess whether the skills of a therapist are required. As such, we disagree with the commenter that this is a new limiting criterion. We also disagree that the proposed regulation text changes do not adequately consider the unique condition of the patient when clarifying coverage requirements. In fact, we believe the proposed regulation text changes at § 409.44(c)(2)(iii) refer more comprehensively than the current regulation text to the patient's unique clinical condition as a criterion for determining whether the complex services which must be provided by a therapist are needed. Regarding the commenter's concern that the proposed regulation text changes newly require that maintenance therapy must be needed in connection with a specific disease, we also disagree. Current regulations at § 409.44(c)(2)(iii) describe that establishing a maintenance program would be covered if the skills of a therapist are needed to provide a safe and effective maintenance program in connection with a specific disease. However, we agree that the words "in connection with the patient's illness or injury" instead of "in connection with a specific disease" would be an improvement to the regulation text and we are making this change in this final rule. We disagree with the commenter that current policy allows maintenance therapy to be covered when the skills of a therapist are needed to ensure the patient's safety OR the skills of a therapist are needed in order to provide a safe and effective maintenance program. We have required in regulation and longstanding manual guidance that the skills of a therapist would be required to ensure both patient safety and effectiveness of a maintenance program for the performance of maintenance therapy to be covered.

We refer the commenter to current regulations at § 409.44(c)(2)(iii) and longstanding manual guidance at 40.2.2 E. in chapter 7 of the Medicare Benefit Policy Manual, CMS Pub. 100–2. Regarding the commenter's concern that current § 409.32(c) mandates the restoration potential of a patient is not the deciding factor in determining whether skilled services are needed, and even if full recovery or medical improvement is not possible, a patient may need skilled services to prevent further deterioration or preserve current capabilities, we reply that we believe the commenter may be misunderstanding the current regulation text at § 409.32(c) or interpreting this out of its proper context. We believe it is important to again note that the emphasis for our therapy coverage criteria is not on the issue of restoration potential per se, but rather on the beneficiary's need for complex services which require the skills of a qualified therapist. Current regulations at § 409.32(c) specify that it is the beneficiary's need for *skilled services* rather than his or her restoration potential that is the deciding factor in evaluating the need for skilled nursing services in the HH setting. A beneficiary's restoration potential has never been a factor at all in identifying those services that constitute skilled *nursing* care. Thus, nursing care can be considered skilled without regard to whether it serves to improve a beneficiary's condition or to maintain the beneficiary's current level of functioning. In fact, as the original version of this regulation's text [as initially codified at 20 CFR § 405.127(b)(2) (40 FR 43897, September 24, 1975)] makes clear, this provision's example of a terminal cancer patient was intended to refer specifically to *nursing* services that can be considered skilled "even though no potential for *rehabilitation* exists" (emphasis added). Longstanding current regulatory language at § 409.44(c) sets out the criteria for skilled therapy (as opposed to the skilled nursing criteria described above) to be a covered service under Medicare's HH benefit. Current regulations specify that HH therapy services are covered based on the inherent complexity of the service which the patient needs, and whether the needed services require the skills of a qualified therapist. Further, current regulations state that HH therapy services are covered if there is an expectation that the patient's condition will improve in a reasonable and predictable timeframe based on the physician's assessment of the

beneficiary's restoration potential and unique medical condition of the patient. Current regulations also allow for therapy coverage when, for safety and effectiveness, the unique medical complexities of the patient require a qualified therapist's skills in the establishment or performance of a therapy maintenance program.

Regarding the commenter's concerns that, should we require improvement as a therapy coverage criteria, we would be applying an arbitrary "rule of thumb" which does not consider the patient's individual condition, and as such, the requirement conflicts with the current regulation at § 409.44, we again assure the commenter that we are not expanding or limiting the coverage of HH therapy. To address the commenter's concerns regarding the potential for claims denials based on "rules of thumb," we assure the commenter that such denials are prohibited.

"Rules of thumb" in the Medicare medical review process are prohibited. Intermediaries must not make denial decisions solely on the reviewer's general inferences about beneficiaries with similar diagnoses or on general data related to utilization. Any "rules of thumb" that would declare a claim not covered solely on the basis of elements, such as, lack of restoration potential, ability to walk a certain number of feet, or degree of stability, is unacceptable without individual review of all pertinent facts to determine if coverage may be justified. Medical denial decisions must be based on a detailed and thorough analysis of the beneficiary's total condition and individual need for care.

Similar instructions have appeared as far back as 1992 in the previous, paper-based manuals (available online at *http://www.cms.gov/Manuals/PBM/ list.asp*), in section 3900.A of the Medicare Intermediary Manual, Part 3 (CMS Pub. 13–3), and in section 214.7 of the Medicare SNF Manual (CMS Pub. 12).

Regarding the comment that the proposed regulation does not define "reasonable and necessary" in a way that clearly provides for coverage of maintenance therapy, we believe the commenter took issue with proposed clarifications surrounding regulations at § 409.44(c)(2)(iv) which state that the amount, frequency, and duration of services must be reasonable. In these revisions we describe that therapy can be considered reasonable and necessary when the criteria for maintenance therapy are met. We believe the commenter suggests we more definitively state that therapy would be

APPENDIX

covered in such a case. We concur, and we will make this change.

Comment: One commenter noted that under a state's approved Medicaid State Plan Amendment, therapies may be authorized as appropriate to maintain function or to slow the rate of decline in function. This commenter therefore requested that we consider whether the proposed rule language should be revised to clarify a potential difference in benefits [under Medicaid versus Medicare] or if revised instructions regarding Conditions of Participation (CoPs) applicability is sufficient. For whatever option we choose, this commenter indicated that we should contemplate using the Medicare rules as the foundation for Medicaid HH program rules as this commenter believes that changes are needed to accommodate the permitted differences in benefits.

Response: We thank the commenter but note such a suggestion is outside the scope of this rule, and the issue for which we solicited comments. We will consider this suggestion in the future as we analyze improvements to the HH PPS.

Comment: Commenters stated that, while they applaud our efforts to better define medical necessity and document therapy services, they were also concerned that the new documentation requirements will be a difficult transition for HHAs, stating that the proposed requirement would require significant time and resources for HHAs to ensure that their therapists and other medical staff are educated and prepared to implement the new requirements into their everyday practices. Consequently, this commenter recommended we provide extensive educational outreach and the commenter asked that we delay implementation of these requirements to provide agencies time to retrain staff.

This commenter also recommended that we elaborate further on provisions of the proposed § 409.44(c)(1), including citing references to resources we used for the phrase "with accepted standards of clinical practice," asking us to indicate that these included resources from professional associations. In addition, this commenter asked that we indicate that the "therapy goals" be established by the qualified therapist in conjunction with the physician. This commenter also requested that we further clarify what we mean by objective measurement of therapy progress by including activities of daily living such as walking, eating, bathing, etc. With respect to § 409.44(c)(2)(i), this commenter asked that we clarify what are considered to be "accepted practice" and "effective treatment." Similar to

other commenters, this commenter requested that we further acknowledge multi-therapy cases and insert language that allows for some type of window for completing the reassessment prior to or after the 13th or 19th therapy visits, stating that the adjustment should be made to account for extenuating circumstances that are outside the control of the qualified therapist. Regarding assistants making clinical notes, this commenter suggested that we change the phrase "job title" to "professional designation" and clarify that written and electronic signatures are acceptable. Some commenters asked that we eliminate § 409.44(c)(2)(i) altogether. Regarding § 409.44(c)(2)(iii), this commenter requested that because "rehabilitative" and "restorative" are not interchangeable, we change our regulations to be consistent throughout, using only the word "rehabilitative." This commenter also asked that we add a sentence to clearly state that the maintenance program must be established by the qualified therapist. With respect to § 409.44(c)(2)(iv), this commenter asked that we elaborate on the phrase "with accepted standards of clinical practice" and highlight the importance of educating caregivers to ensure patients receive the appropriate level of care. The commenter also requested that we delay implementation of these requirements until April 2011 to allow time for providers to transition.

Response: We thank the commenter for the suggested clarifications and we have adopted the suggested clarifications with some exceptions. We have retained the language in our current regulatory text at § 409.44(c)(2)(iii) which presently mandates that for therapy to be covered, there must be an expectation that the beneficiary's condition will improve materially in a reasonable (and generally predictable) period of time based on the physician's assessment of the beneficiary's restoration potential and medical condition. Typically, we use the term "rehabilitative" to describe services provided by therapists. In the regulation text, we describe the physician's assessment and therefore we believe the "restorative" terminology is appropriate. However, we will finalize additional changes to the proposed regulation text to achieve more consistency in the usage of these terms. As described in an earlier comment, we have adopted the commenter's request for flexibility associated with the 13th and 19th visit. We believe that clarifications regarding electronic signatures are better addressed in manual guidance. Finally, we will

implement this provision beginning April 2011.

Comment: Some commenters urged CMS to transform the HH PPS therapy reimbursement model to one based on clinical outcomes and skill improvement. A commenter urged CMS to adopt tests for clinicians, which assess the clinician's abilities.

Response: We thank the commenter for these suggestions. As we described in earlier comment responses, section 3131(d) of the Affordable Care Act requires CMS to conduct a study on costs involved with providing HH services for patients with high severity of illness, including analysis of potential revisions to outlier payments to better reflect costs of treating Medicare beneficiaries and analyze other HH PPS issues determined by the Secretary. We intend to use this opportunity to assess a variety of HH PPS issues, including our current HH PPS therapy threshold reimbursement.

Comment: A commenter suggested that CMS consider making access to physician-ordered medically necessary music therapy as a covered service.

Response: We thank the commenter but note that Congress would need to enact legislation in order to cover music therapy services under Medicare's HH benefit, as they are not currently covered HH services as defined in section 1861(m) of the Act.

Comment: Commenters provided feedback regarding our plans to revise G-codes to reflect greater detail in the reporting of skilled nursing and therapy services. Many commenters requested more time (6 months to a year or more) be allowed before these new and revised codes become effective, so as to give more time for CMS to provide direction to HHAs and thus provide time for agencies to train staff and modify data collection systems to accommodate these coding changes. Another commenter questioned the lead-time to establish new G-codes, stating that it would be impossible for all necessary program changes to be made to all vendor software within three months. This commenter requested that CMS postpone the new and revised G-codes until 2012 to give agencies and vendors time to reprogram the requirements. The commenter also suggested that the types of descriptions of the codes identified suggest that CMS wants to use the codes to determine medically reasonable and necessary care rather than doing actual medical review of patient clinical records. The commenter noted that 60 to 75 percent of claims in which the appeals are taken to the administrative law judge level are reversed and suggested that we already have an issue with our medical review and program integrity units that would be further exacerbated by the proposed G-codes.

Response: It is important to note that we provided the information on the new G-codes to the industry as a pre-notification of our intention to collect additional information on the claim. The implementation of this provision will be issued in an administrative change notice. We note that in describing our plans in the proposed rule published on July 23, 2010, we intended to provided the industry with early information so that they could begin planning for this change at that time. We currently plan to implement this reporting requirement in January 2011. However, we thank the commenter, and we will consider this suggestion.

Comment: Commenters expressed concern regarding G-code 6, stating that it has combined two dissimilar activities and should be split to avoid confusion, resulting in possible erroneous data. Specifically, commenters indicated that a G-code for services for the management and evaluation of the plan of care should be separate from a G-code for the services for the observation and assessment of a patient's condition while a patient's treatment is stabilized.

Response: We concur with this suggestion and will adopt the separate G-codes.

Comment: Some commenters asked that in revising and adding G-codes for the reporting of HH services, CMS should also consider creating codes to differentiate between the services provided by a registered nurse (RN) and a licensed practical nurse (LPN).

Response: We thank the commenters for this suggestion and will consider their recommendation in future rulemaking.

In summary, we thank the many commenters for their thoughtful and comprehensive suggestions. After considering these comments, we will finalize the proposed therapy coverage clarifications with several changes. We will delay the implementation of the therapy provisions until April 1, 2011, to allow agencies more transition time. We will finalize exceptions to the 13th and 19th qualified therapy visit requirement to provide some flexibility associated with patients in rural areas, patients receiving more than 1 therapy discipline, and documented exceptional circumstances which would preclude the therapist from performing the needed 13th or 19th visit. We have made regulatory text changes to remove confusing scenarios associated with maintenance therapy, which led commenters to believe that maintenance

therapy was a dependent service. We will finalize numerous other regulation text changes to clarify that these changes do not impose new limitations on the coverage of maintenance therapy. The changes include clarifications that when the criteria for maintenance therapy is met, a qualified therapist would be assessing the effectiveness of the therapy provided, rather than the patient's progress. Other changes include the removal of definitions of rehabilitative therapy which were confusing to commenters, and other miscellaneous regulation text clarifications which were suggested and we believe improve the clarity of the regulation text.

C. Outlier Policy

1. Background

Section 1895(b)(5) of the Act allows for the provision of an addition or adjustment to the national standardized 60-day case-mix and wage-adjusted episode payment amounts in the case of episodes that incur unusually high costs due to patient HH care needs. Prior to the enactment of the Affordable Care Act in March 2010, this section stipulated that total outlier payments could not exceed 5 percent of total projected or estimated HH payments in a given year. Under the HH PPS, outlier payments are made for episodes for which the estimated costs exceed a threshold amount. The wage adjusted fixed dollar loss (FDL) amount represents the amount of loss that an agency must absorb before an episode becomes eligible for outlier payments. As outlined in our FY 2000 HH PPS final rule (65 FR 41188 through 41190), Medicare provided for outlier payments not to exceed 5 percent of total payments and adjusted the payment rates accordingly.

2. Regulatory Update

In our November 10, 2009 HH PPS final rule for CY 2010 (74 FR 58080 through 58087), we explained that our analysis revealed excessive growth in outlier payments in discrete areas of the country. Despite program integrity efforts associated with excessive outlier payments in targeted areas of the country, we discovered that outlier expenditures exceeded the 5 percent statutory limit. Consequently, we assessed the appropriateness of taking action to curb outlier abuse.

In order to mitigate possible billing vulnerabilities associated with excessive outlier payments, and to adhere to our statutory limit on outlier payments, we adopted an outlier policy of an agency-level cap on outlier payments at 10

percent of the agency's total payments, in concert with a reduced FDL ratio of 0.67. This policy resulted in a projected target outlier pool of approximately 2.5 percent (the previous outlier pool target was 5 percent of total HH expenditures). For CY 2010, we first returned 5 percent back into the national standardized 60-day episode rates, the national per-visit rates, the LUPA add-on payment amount, and the NRS conversion factor. Then, we reduced the CY 2010 rates by 2.5 percent to account for the new outlier pool targeted to 2.5 percent. This revised outlier policy was adopted for CY 2010 only.

3. Statutory Update

Section 3131(b)(1) of the Affordable Care Act amended section 1895(b)(3)(C) of the Act, "Adjustment for outliers," to state, "The Secretary shall reduce the standard prospective payment amount (or amounts) under this paragraph applicable to HH services furnished during a period by such proportion as will result in an aggregate reduction in payments for the period equal to 5 percent of the total payments estimated to be made based on the prospective payment system under this subsection for the period." In addition, section 3131(b)(2) of the Affordable Care Act amended section 1895(b)(5) of the Act by redesignating the existing language as section 1895(b)(5)(A) of the Act, and revising it to state that the Secretary, "may provide for an addition or adjustment to the payment amount otherwise made in the case of outliers because of unusual variations in the type or amount of medically necessary care. The total amount of the additional payments or payment adjustments made under this paragraph with respect to a fiscal year or year may not exceed 2.5 percent of the total payments projected or estimated to be made based on the prospective payment system under this subsection in that year." As such, our HH PPS outlier policy must reduce payment rates by 5 percent, and target up to 2.5 percent of total estimated HH PPS payments to be paid as outlier payments. We will first return the 2.5 percent held for the target CY 2010 outlier pool to the national standardized 60-day episode rates, the national per-visit rates, the LUPA add-on payment amount, and the NRS conversion factor for CY 2010. We will then reduce these rates by 5 percent as required by section 1895(b)(3)(C) of the Act, as amended by section 3131(b)(1) of the Affordable Care Act. For CY 2011 and subsequent calendar years, the total amount of the additional payments or payment adjustments made may not exceed 2.5 percent of the total payments projected

Title 42--Public Health

CHAPTER IV--HEALTH CARE FINANCING ADMINISTRATION, DEPARTMENT OF HEALTH AND HUMAN SERVICES

PART 484--CONDITIONS OF PARTICIPATION: HOME HEALTH AGENCIES

www.access.gpo.gov/nara/cfr/waisidx_99/42cfr484_99.html

Sec. 484.4 Personnel qualifications.

Staff required to meet the conditions set forth in this part are staff who meet the qualifications specified in this section. Administrator, home health agency. A person who:
   (a) Is a licensed physician; or
   (b) Is a registered nurse; or
   (c) Has training and experience in health service administration and at least 1 year of supervisory or administrative experience in home health care or related health programs.

Audiologist. A person who:
   (a) Meets the education and experience requirements for a Certificate of Clinical Competence in audiology granted by the American Speech-Language-Hearing Association; or
   (b) Meets the educational requirements for certification and is in the process of accumulating the supervised experience required for certification.

Home health aide. Effective for services furnished after August 14, 1990, a person who has successfully completed a State-established or other training program that meets the requirements of Sec. 484.36(a) and a competency evaluation program or State licensure program that meets the requirements of Sec. 484.36 (b) or (e), or a competency evaluation program or State licensure program that meets the requirements of Sec. 484.36 (b) or (e). An individual is not considered to have completed a training and competency evaluation program, or a competency evaluation program if, since the individual's most recent completion of this program(s), there has been a continuous period of 24 consecutive months during none of which the individual furnished services described in Sec. 409.40 of this chapter for compensation.

Occupational therapist. A person who:

(a) Is a graduate of an occupational therapy curriculum accredited jointly by the Committee on Allied Health Education and Accreditation of the American Medical Association and the American Occupational Therapy Association; or

(b) Is eligible for the National Registration Examination of the American Occupational Therapy Association; or

(c) Has 2 years of appropriate experience as an occupational therapist, and has achieved a satisfactory grade on a proficiency examination conducted, approved, or sponsored by the U.S. Public Health Service, except that such determinations of proficiency do not apply with respect to persons initially licensed by a State or seeking initial qualification as an occupational therapist after December 31, 1977.

Occupational therapy assistant. A person who:

(a) Meets the requirements for certification as an occupational therapy assistant established by the American Occupational Therapy Association; or

(b) Has 2 years of appropriate experience as an occupational therapy assistant, and has achieved a satisfactory grade on a proficiency examination conducted, approved, or sponsored by the U.S. Public Health Service, except that such determinations of proficiency do not apply with respect to persons initially licensed by a State or seeking initial qualification as an occupational therapy assistant after December 31, 1977.

Physical therapist. A person who is licensed as a physical therapist by the State in which practicing, and

(a) Has graduated from a physical therapy curriculum approved by:

(1) The American Physical Therapy Association, or

(2) The Committee on Allied Health Education and Accreditation of the American Medical Association, or

(3) The Council on Medical Education of the American Medical Association and the American Physical Therapy Association; or

(b) Prior to January 1, 1966,

(1) Was admitted to membership by the American Physical Therapy Association, or

(2) Was admitted to registration by the American Registry of Physical Therapist, or

(3) Has graduated from a physical therapy curriculum in a 4-year college or university approved by a State department of education; or

(c) Has 2 years of appropriate experience as a physical therapist, and has achieved a satisfactory grade on a proficiency examination conducted, approved, or sponsored by the U.S. Public Health Service except that such determinations of proficiency do not apply with respect to persons initially licensed by a State or seeking qualification as a physical therapist after December 31, 1977; or

(d) Was licensed or registered prior to January 1, 1966, and prior to January 1, 1970, had 15 years of full-time experience in the treatment of illness or injury through the practice of physical therapy in which services were rendered under the order and direction of attending and referring doctors of medicine or osteopathy; or

(e) If trained outside the United States,

(1) Was graduated since 1928 from a physical therapy curriculum approved in the country in which the curriculum was located and in which there is a member organization of the World Confederation for Physical Therapy.

(2) Meets the requirements for membership in a member organization of the World Confederation for Physical Therapy,

Physical therapy assistant. A person who is licensed as a physical therapy assistant, if applicable, by the State in which practicing, and

(1) Has graduated from a 2-year college-level program approved by the American Physical Therapy Association; or

(2) Has 2 years of appropriate experience as a physical therapy assistant, and has achieved a satisfactory grade on a proficiency examination conducted, approved, or sponsored by the U.S. Public Health Service, except that these determinations of proficiency do not apply with respect to persons initially licensed by a State or seeking initial qualification as a physical therapy assistant after December 31, 1977.

Physician. A doctor of medicine, osteophathy or podiatry legally authorized to practice medicine and surgery by the State in which such function or action is performed.

Practical (vocational) nurse. A person who is licensed as a practical (vocational) nurse by the State in which practicing.

Public health nurse. A registered nurse who has completed a baccalaureate degree program approved by the National League for Nursing for public health nursing preparation or postregistered nurse study that includes content approved by the National League for Nursing for public health nursing preparation.

Registered nurse (RN). A graduate of an approved school of professional nursing, who is licensed as a registered nurse by the State in which practicing.

Social work assistant. A person who:

(1) Has a baccalaureate degree in social work, psychology, sociology, or other field related to social work, and has had at least 1 year of social work experience in a health care setting; or

(2) Has 2 years of appropriate experience as a social work assistant, and has achieved a satisfactory grade on a proficiency examination conducted, approved, or sponsored by the U.S. Public Health Service, except that these determinations of proficiency do not apply with respect to persons initially licensed by a State or seeking initial qualification as a social work assistant after December 31, 1977.

Social worker. A person who has a master's degree from a school of social work accredited by the Council on Social Work Education, and has 1 year of social work experience in a health care setting.

Speech-language pathologist. A person who:

(1) Meets the education and experience requirements for a Certificate of Clinical Competence in (speech pathology or audiology) granted by the American Speech-Language-Hearing Association; or

(2) Meets the educational requirements for certification and is in the process of accumulating the supervised experience required for certification.

[54 FR 33367, August 14, 1989, as amended at 56 FR 32973, July 18, 1991]

Sec. 484.10 Condition of participation: Patient rights.

The patient has the right to be informed of his or her rights. The HHA must protect and promote the exercise of these rights.

(a) Standard: Notice of rights. (1) The HHA must provide the patient with a written notice of the patient's rights in advance of furnishing care to the patient or during the initial evaluation visit before the initiation of treatment.

(2) The HHA must maintain documentation showing that it has complied with the requirements of this section.

(b) Standard: Exercise of rights and respect for property and person. (1) The patient has the right to exercise his or her rights as a patient of the HHA.

(2) The patient's family or guardian may exercise the patient's rights when the patient has been judged incompetent.

(3) The patient has the right to have his or her property treated with respect.

(4) The patient has the right to voice grievances regarding treatment or care that is (or fails to be) furnished, or regarding the lack of respect for property by anyone who is furnishing services on behalf of the HHA and must not be subjected to discrimination or reprisal for doing so.

(5) The HHA must investigate complaints made by a patient or the patient's family or guardian regarding treatment or care that is (or fails to be) furnished, or regarding the lack of respect for the patient's property by anyone furnishing services on behalf of the HHA, and must document both the existence of the complaint and the resolution of the complaint.

(c) Standard: Right to be informed and to participate in planning care and treatment. (1) The patient has the right to be informed, in advance about the care to be furnished, and of any changes in the care to be furnished.

(i) The HHA must advise the patient in advance of the disciplines that will furnish care, and the frequency of visits proposed to be furnished.

(ii) The HHA must advise the patient in advance of any change in the plan of care before the change is made.

(2) The patient has the right to participate in the planning of the care.

(i) The HHA must advise the patient in advance of the right to participate in planning the care or treatment and in planning changes in the care or treatment.

(ii) The HHA complies with the requirements of subpart I of part 489 of this chapter relating to maintaining written policies and procedures regarding advance directives. The HHA must inform and distribute written information to the patient, in advance, concerning its policies on advance directives, including a description of applicable State law. The HHA may furnish advance directives information to a patient at the time of the first home visit, as long as the information is furnished before care is provided.

(d) Standard: Confidentiality of medical records. The patient has the right to confidentiality of the clinical records maintained by the HHA. The HHA must advise the patient of the agency's policies and procedures regarding disclosure of clinical records.

(e) Standard: Patient liability for payment. (1) The patient has the right to be advised, before care is initiated, of the extent to which payment for the HHA services may be expected from Medicare or other sources, and the extent to which payment may be required from the patient. Before the care is initiated, the HHA must inform the patient, orally and in writing, of--

(i) The extent to which payment may be expected from Medicare, Medicaid, or any other Federally funded or aided program known to the HHA;

(ii) The charges for services that will not be covered by Medicare; and

(iii) The charges that the individual may have to pay.

(2) The patient has the right to be advised orally and in writing of any changes in the information provided in accordance with paragraph
(e)(1) of this section when they occur. The HHA must advise the patient of these changes orally and in writing as soon as possible, but no later than 30 calendar days from the date that the HHA becomes aware of a change.

(f) Standard: Home health hotline. The patient has the right to be advised of the availability of the toll-free HHA hotline in the State. When the agency accepts the patient for treatment or care, the HHA must advise the patient in writing of the telephone number of the home health hotline established by the State, the hours of its operation, and that the purpose of the hotline is to receive complaints or questions about local HHAs. The patient also has the right to use this hotline to lodge complaints concerning the implementation of the advance directives requirements.

[54 FR 33367, August 14, 1989, as amended at 56 FR 32973, July 18, 1991; 57 FR 8203, Mar. 6, 1992; 60 FR 33293, June 27, 1995]

Sec. 484.12 Condition of participation: Compliance with Federal, State, and local laws, disclosure and ownership information, and accepted professional standards and principles.

(a) Standard: Compliance with Federal, State, and local laws and regulations. The HHA and its staff must operate and furnish services in compliance with all applicable Federal, State, and local laws and regulations. If State or applicable local law provides for the licensure of HHAs, an agency not subject to licensure is approved by the licensing authority as meeting the standards established for licensure.

(b) Standard: Disclosure of ownership and management information. The HHA must comply with the requirements of Part 420, Subpart C of this chapter. The HHA also must disclose the following information to the State survey agency at the time of the HHA's initial request for certification, for each survey, and at the time of any change in ownership or management:

(1) The name and address of all persons with an ownership or control interest in the HHA as defined in Secs. 420.201, 420.202, and 420.206 of this chapter.

(2) The name and address of each person who is an officer, a director, an agent or a managing employee of the HHA as defined in Secs. 420.201, 420.202, and 420.206 of this chapter.

(3) The name and address of the corporation, association, or other company that is responsible for the management of the HHA, and the name and address of the chief executive officer and the chairman of the board of directors of that corporation, association, or other company responsible for the management of the HHA.

(c) Standard: Compliance with accepted professional standards and principles. The HHA and its staff must comply with accepted professional standards and principles that apply to professionals furnishing services in an HHA.

Sec. 484.18 Condition of participation: Acceptance of patients, plan of care, and medical supervision.

Patients are accepted for treatment on the basis of a reasonable expectation that the patient's medical, nursing, and social needs can be met adequately by the agency in the patient's place of residence. Care follows a written plan of care established and periodically reviewed by a doctor of medicine, osteopathy, or podiatric medicine.

(a) Standard: Plan of care. The plan of care developed in consultation with the agency staff covers all pertinent diagnoses, including mental status, types of services and equipment required, frequency of visits, prognosis, rehabilitation potential, functional limitations, activities permitted, nutritional requirements, medications and treatments, any safety measures to protect against injury, instructions for timely discharge or referral, and any other appropriate items. If a physician refers a patient under a plan of care that cannot be completed until after an evaluation visit, the physician is consulted to approve additions or modifications to the original plan. Orders for therapy services include the specific procedures and modalities to be used and the amount, frequency, and duration. The therapist and other agency personnel participate in developing the plan of care.

(b) Standard: Periodic review of plan of care. The total plan of care is reviewed by the attending physician and HHA personnel as often as the severity of the patient's condition requires, but at least once every 62 days. Agency professional staff promptly alert the physician to any changes that suggest a need to alter the plan of care.

(c) Standard: Conformance with physician orders. Drugs and treatments are administered by agency staff only as ordered by the physician. Verbal orders are put in writing and signed and dated with the date of receipt by the registered nurse or qualified therapist (as defined in Sec. 484.4 of this chapter) responsible for furnishing or supervising the ordered services. Verbal orders are only accepted by personnel authorized to do so by applicable State and Federal laws and regulations as well as by the HHA's internal policies.

[54 FR 33367, August 14, 1989, as amended at 56 FR 32974, July 18, 1991; 64 FR 3784, Jan. 25, 1999]

Sec. 484.20 Condition of participation: Reporting OASIS information.

HHAs must electronically report all OASIS data collected in accordance with Sec. 484.55.

(a) Standard: Encoding OASIS data. The HHA must encode and be capable of transmitting OASIS data for each agency patient within 7 days of completing an OASIS data set.

(b) Standard: Accuracy of encoded OASIS data. The encoded OASIS data must accurately reflect the patient's status at the time of assessment.

(c) Standard: Transmittal of OASIS data. The HHA must--

(1) Electronically transmit accurate, completed, encoded and locked OASIS data for each patient to the State agency or HCFA OASIS contractor at least monthly;

(2) For all assessments completed in the previous month, transmit OASIS data in a format that meets the requirements of paragraph (d) of this section;

(3) Successfully transmit test data to the State agency or HCFA OASIS contractor beginning March 26, 1999, and no later than April 26, 1999; and

(4) Transmit data using electronic communications software that provides a direct telephone connection from the HHA to the State agency or HCFA OASIS contractor.

(d) Standard: Data Format. The HHA must encode and transmit data using the software available from HCFA or software that conforms to HCFA standard electronic record layout, edit specifications, and data dictionary, and that includes the required OASIS data set.

[64 FR 3763, Jan. 25, 1999]

Sec. 484.32 Condition of participation: Therapy services.

Any therapy services offered by the HHA directly or under arrangement are given by a qualified therapist or by a qualified therapy assistant under the supervision of a qualified therapist and in accordance with the plan of care. The qualified therapist assists the physician in evaluating level of function, helps develop the plan of care (revising it as necessary), prepares clinical and progress notes, advises and consults with the family and other agency personnel, and participates in in-service programs.

(a) Standard: Supervision of physical therapy assistant and occupational therapy assistant. Services furnished by a qualified physical therapy assistant or qualified occupational therapy assistant may be furnished under the supervision of a qualified physical or occupational therapist. A physical therapy assistant or occupational therapy assistant performs services planned, delegated, and supervised by the therapist, assists in preparing clinical notes and progress reports, and participates in educating the patient and family, and in in-service programs.

(b) Standard: Supervision of speech therapy services. Speech therapy services are furnished only by or under supervision of a qualified speech pathologist or audiologist.

[54 FR 33367, August 14, 1989, as amended at 56 FR 32974, July 18, 1991]

Sec. 484.48 Condition of participation: Clinical records.

A clinical record containing pertinent past and current findings in accordance with accepted professional standards is maintained for every patient receiving home health services. In addition to the plan of care, the record contains appropriate identifying information; name of physician; drug, dietary, treatment, and activity orders; signed and dated clinical and progress notes; copies of summary reports sent to the attending physician; and a discharge summary. The HHA must inform the attending physician of the availability of a discharge summary. The discharge summary must be sent to the attending physician upon request and must include the patient's medical and health status at discharge.

(a) Standards: Retention of records. Clinical records are retained for 5 years after the month the cost report to which the records apply is filed with the intermediary, unless State law stipulates a longer period of time. Policies provide for retention even if the HHA discontinues operations. If a patient is transferred to another health facility, a copy of the record or abstract is sent with the patient.

(b) Standards: Protection of records. Clinical record information is safe-guarded against loss or unauthorized use. Written procedures govern use and removal of records and the conditions for release of information. Patient's written consent is required for release of information not authorized by law.

[54 FR 33367, Aug. 14, 1989, as amended at 60 FR 65498, Dec. 20, 1994]

Sec. 484.55 Condition of participation: Comprehensive assessment of patients.

Each patient must receive, and an HHA must provide, a patient-specific, comprehensive assessment that accurately reflects the patient's current health status and includes information that may be used to demonstrate the patient's progress toward achievement of desired outcomes. The comprehensive assessment must identify the patient's continuing need for home care and meet the patient's medical, nursing, rehabilitative, social, and discharge planning needs. For Medicare beneficiaries, the HHA must verify the patient's eligibility for the Medicare home health benefit including homebound status, both at the time of the initial assessment visit and at the time of the comprehensive assessment. The comprehensive assessment must also incorporate the use of the current version of the Outcome and Assessment Information Set (OASIS) items, using the language and groupings of the OASIS items, as specified by the Secretary.

(a) Standard: Initial assessment visit. (1) A registered nurse must conduct an initial assessment visit to determine the immediate care and support needs of the patient; and, for Medicare patients, to determine eligibility for the Medicare home health benefit, including homebound status. The initial assessment visit must be held either within 48 hours of referral, or within 48 hours of the patient's return home, or on the physician-ordered start of care date.

(2) When rehabilitation therapy service (speech language pathology, physical therapy, or occupational therapy) is the only service ordered by the physician, and if the need for that service establishes program eligibility, the initial assessment visit may be made by the appropriate rehabilitation skilled professional.

(b) Standard: Completion of the comprehensive assessment. (1) The comprehensive assessment must be completed in a timely manner, consistent with the patient's immediate needs, but no later than 5 calendar days after the start of care.

(2) Except as provided in paragraph (b)(3) of this section, a registered nurse must complete the comprehensive assessment and for Medicare patients, determine eligibility for the Medicare home health benefit, including homebound status.

(3) When physical therapy, speech-language pathology, or occupational therapy is the only service ordered by the physician, a physical therapist, speech-language pathologist or occupational therapist may complete the comprehensive assessment, and for Medicare patients, determine eligibility for the Medicare home health benefit, including homebound status. The occupational therapist may complete the comprehensive assessment if the need for occupational therapy establishes program eligibility.

(c) Standard: Drug regimen review. The comprehensive assessment must include a review of all medications the patient is currently using in order to identify any potential adverse effects and drug reactions, including ineffective drug therapy, significant side effects, significant drug interactions, duplicate drug therapy, and noncompliance with drug therapy.

(d) Standard: Update of the comprehensive assessment. The comprehensive assessment must be updated and revised (including the administration of the OASIS) as frequently as the patient's condition warrants due to a major decline or improvement in the patient's health status, but not less frequently than--

(1) Every second calendar month beginning with the start of care date;

(2) Within 48 hours of the patient's return to the home from a hospital admission of 24 hours or more for any reason other than diagnostic tests;

(3) At discharge.

(e) Standard: Incorporation of OASIS data items. The OASIS data items determined by the Secretary must be incorporated into the HHA's own assessment and must include: clinical record items, demographics and patient history, living arrangements, supportive assistance, sensory status, integumentary status, respiratory status, elimination status, neuro/emotional/behavioral status, activities of daily living, medications, equipment management, emergent care, and data items collected at inpatient facility admission or discharge only.

[64 FR 3784, Jan. 25, 1999]

OMB #0938-0760

Expiration date 7/31/2012

According to the Paperwork Reduction Act of 1995, no persons are required to respond to a collection of information unless it displays a valid OMB control number. The valid OMB control number for this information collection instrument is 0938-0760. The time required to complete this information collection is estimated to average 0.7 minutes per response, including the time to review instructions, search existing data resources, gather the data needed, and complete and review the information collection. If you have comments concerning this form, please write to: CMS, 7500 Security Boulevard, Attn: PRA Reports Clearance Officer, Baltimore, Maryland 21244-1850.

Home Health Patient Tracking Sheet

(M0010) C M S Certification Number: _ _ _ _ _ _ _

(M0014) Branch State: _ _

(M0016) Branch I D Number: _ _ _ _ _ _ _ _ _ _

(M0018) National Provider Identifier (N P I) for the attending physician who has signed the plan of care:

_ _ _ _ _ _ _ _ _ _   ☐ **UK – Unknown or Not Available**

(M0020) Patient I D Number: _ _ _ _ _ _ _ _ _ _ _ _ _ _ _ _ _ _ _

(M0030) Start of Care Date: _ _ / _ _ / _ _ _ _
month / day / year

(M0032) Resumption of Care Date: _ _ / _ _ / _ _ _ _   ☐ **NA - Not Applicable**
month / day / year

(M0040) Patient Name:

_ _ _ _ _ _ _ _ _ _ _ _ _ _ _ _ _ _ _ _ _ _ _ _ _ _ _   _ _ _
(First)   (M I) (Last)   (Suffix)

(M0050) Patient State of Residence: _ _

(M0060) Patient Zip Code: _ _ _ _ _ _ _ _ _

(M0063) Medicare Number: _ _ _ _ _ _ _ _ _ _ _ _   ☐ **NA – No Medicare**
(including suffix)

(M0064) Social Security Number: _ _ _ - _ _ - _ _ _ _   ☐ **UK – Unknown or Not Available**

(M0065) Medicaid Number: _ _ _ _ _ _ _ _ _ _ _ _ _   ☐ **NA – No Medicaid**

(M0066) Birth Date: _ _ / _ _ / _ _ _ _
month / day / year

(M0069) Gender:

☐   1 - Male
☐   2 - Female

(M0140) Race/Ethnicity: (Mark all that apply.)

☐   1 - American Indian or Alaska Native
☐   2 - Asian
☐   3 - Black or African-American
☐   4 - Hispanic or Latino
☐   5 - Native Hawaiian or Pacific Islander
☐   6 - White

OASIS-C: All Items
Centers for Medicare & Medicaid Services   August 2009   Page 1 of 24

APPENDIX

OMB #0938-0760

Expiration date 7/31/2012

(M0150) Current Payment Sources for Home Care: (Mark all that apply.)

- ☐ 0 - None; no charge for current services
- ☐ 1 - Medicare (traditional fee-for-service)
- ☐ 2 - Medicare (HMO/managed care/Advantage plan)
- ☐ 3 - Medicaid (traditional fee-for-service)
- ☐ 4 - Medicaid (HMO/managed care)
- ☐ 5 - Workers' compensation
- ☐ 6 - Title programs (e.g., Title III, V, or XX)
- ☐ 7 - Other government (e.g., TriCare, VA, etc.)
- ☐ 8 - Private insurance
- ☐ 9 - Private HMO/managed care
- ☐ 10 - Self-pay
- ☐ 11 - Other (specify) _____
- ☐ UK - Unknown

APPENDIX

OMB #0938-0760

Expiration date 7/31/2012

Outcome and Assessment Information Set
Items to be Used at Specific Time Points

Start of Care -- Start of care—further visits planned	M0010-M0030, M0040- M0150, M1000-M1036, M1100-M1242, M1300-M1302, M1306, M1308-M1324, M1330-M1350, M1400, M1410, M1600-M1730, M1740-M1910, M2000, M2002, M2010, M2020-M2250
Resumption of Care -- Resumption of care (after inpatient stay)	M0032, M0080-M0110, M1000-M1036, M1100-M1242, M1300-M1302, M1306, M1308-M1324, M1330-M1350, M1400, M1410, M1600-M1730, M1740-M1910, M2000, M2002, M2010, M2020-M2250

Follow-Up --
  Recertification (follow-up) assessment
  Other follow-up assessment
	M0080-M0100, M0110, M1020-M1030, M1200, M1242, M1306, M1308, M1322-M1324, M1330-M1350, M1400, M1610, M1620, M1630, M1810-M1840, M1850, M1860, M2030, M2200

Transfer to an Inpatient Facility-------------------------------
  Transferred to an inpatient facility—patient not discharged from an agency
  Transferred to an inpatient facility—patient discharged from agency
	M0080-M0100, M1040-M1055, M1500, M1510, M2004, M2015, M2300-M2410, M2430-M2440, M0903, M0906

Discharge from Agency — Not to an Inpatient Facility
  Death at home--
  Discharge from agency---------------------------------------
	M0080-M0100, M0903, M0906
	M0080-M0100, M1040-M1055, M1230, M1242, M1306-M1350, M1400-M1620, M1700-M1720, M1740, M1745, M1800-M1890, M2004, M2015-M2030, M2100-M2110, M2300-M2420, M0903, M0906

CLINICAL RECORD ITEMS

(M0080) Discipline of Person Completing Assessment:

☐ 1-RN   ☐ 2-PT   ☐ 3-SLP/ST   ☐ 4-OT

(M0090) Date Assessment Completed: _ _ /_ _ /_ _ _ _

month / day / year

(M0100) This Assessment is Currently Being Completed for the Following Reason:

Start/Resumption of Care
☐   1 – Start of care—further visits planned
☐   3 – Resumption of care (after inpatient stay)

Follow-Up
☐   4 – Recertification (follow-up) reassessment [*Go to M0110*]
☐   5 – Other follow-up [*Go to M0110*]

Transfer to an Inpatient Facility
☐   6 – Transferred to an inpatient facility—patient not discharged from agency [*Go to M1040*]
☐   7 – Transferred to an inpatient facility—patient discharged from agency [*Go to M1040*]

Discharge from Agency — Not to an Inpatient Facility
☐   8 – Death at home [*Go to M0903*]
☐   9 – Discharge from agency [*Go to M1040*]

OASIS-C: All Items
Centers for Medicare & Medicaid Services   August 2009   Page 3 of 24

OMB #0938-0760

Expiration date 7/31/2012

(M0102) **Date of Physician-ordered Start of Care (Resumption of Care):** If the physician indicated a specific start of care (resumption of care) date when the patient was referred for home health services, record the date specified.

＿＿/＿＿/＿＿＿＿　　　*[Go to M0110, if date entered]*
month / day / year

☐　NA –No specific SOC date ordered by physician

(M0104) **Date of Referral:** Indicate the date that the written or verbal referral for initiation or resumption of care was received by the HHA.

＿＿/＿＿/＿＿＿＿
month / day / year

(M0110) **Episode Timing:** Is the Medicare home health payment episode for which this assessment will define a case mix group an "early" episode or a "later" episode in the patient's current sequence of adjacent Medicare home health payment episodes?

☐　1　-　Early

☐　2　-　Later

☐　UK　-　Unknown

☐　NA　-　Not Applicable:　No Medicare case mix group to be defined by this assessment.

PATIENT HISTORY AND DIAGNOSES

(M1000) From which of the following **Inpatient Facilities** was the patient discharged <u>during the past 14 days</u>? **(Mark all that apply.)**

☐　1　-　Long-term nursing facility (NF)

☐　2　-　Skilled nursing facility (SNF / TCU)

☐　3　-　Short-stay acute hospital (IPP S)

☐　4　-　Long-term care hospital (LTCH)

☐　5　-　Inpatient rehabilitation hospital or unit (IRF)

☐　6　-　Psychiatric hospital or unit

☐　7　-　Other (specify) _____

☐　NA　-　Patient was not discharged from an inpatient facility *[Go to M1016]*

(M1005) **Inpatient Discharge Date** (most recent):

＿＿/＿＿/＿＿＿＿
month / day / year

☐　UK　-　Unknown

APPENDIX

OMB #0938-0760

Expiration date 7/31/2012

(M1010) List each **Inpatient Diagnosis** and ICD-9-C M code at the level of highest specificity for only those conditions treated during an inpatient stay within the last 14 days (no E-codes, or V-codes):

Inpatient Facility Diagnosis	ICD-9-C M Code
a. _____	— — — . — —
b. _____	— — — . — —
c. _____	— — — . — —
d. _____	— — — . — —
e. _____	— — — . — —
f. _____	— — — . — —

(M1012) List each **Inpatient Procedure** and the associated ICD-9-C M procedure code relevant to the plan of care.

Inpatient Procedure	Procedure Code
a. _____	— — . — —
b. _____	— — . — —
c. _____	— — . — —
d. _____	— — . — —

☐ NA - Not applicable

☐ UK - Unknown

(M1016) **Diagnoses Requiring Medical or Treatment Regimen Change Within Past 14 Days:** List the patient's Medical Diagnoses and ICD-9-C M codes at the level of highest specificity for those conditions requiring changed medical or treatment regimen within the past 14 days (no surgical, E-codes, or V-codes):

Changed Medical Regimen Diagnosis	ICD-9-C M Code
a. _____	— — — . — —
b. _____	— — — . — —
c. _____	— — — . — —
d. _____	— — — . — —
e. _____	— — — . — —
f. _____	— — — . — —

☐ NA - Not applicable (no medical or treatment regimen changes within the past 14 days)

(M1018) **Conditions Prior to Medical or Treatment Regimen Change or Inpatient Stay Within Past 14 Days**: If this patient experienced an inpatient facility discharge or change in medical or treatment regimen within the past 14 days, indicate any conditions which existed <u>prior to</u> the inpatient stay or change in medical or treatment regimen. **(Mark all that apply.)**

☐ 1 - Urinary incontinence

☐ 2 - Indwelling/suprapubic catheter

☐ 3 - Intractable pain

☐ 4 - Impaired decision-making

☐ 5 - Disruptive or socially inappropriate behavior

☐ 6 - Memory loss to the extent that supervision required

☐ 7 - None of the above

☐ NA - No inpatient facility discharge <u>and</u> no change in medical or treatment regimen in past 14 days

☐ UK - Unknown

APPENDIX

OMB #0938-0760   Expiration date 7/31/2012

(M1020/1022/1024)   Diagnoses, Symptom Control, and Payment Diagnoses: List each diagnosis for which the patient is receiving home care (Column 1) and enter its ICD-9-C M code at the level of highest specificity (no surgical/procedure codes) (Column 2). Diagnoses are listed in the order that best reflect the seriousness of each condition and support the disciplines and services provided. Rate the degree of symptom control for each condition (Column 2). Choose one value that represents the degree of symptom control appropriate for each diagnosis: V-codes (for M1020 or M1022) or E-codes (for M1022 only) may be used. ICD-9-C M sequencing requirements must be followed if multiple coding is indicated for any diagnoses. If a V-code is reported in place of a case mix diagnosis, then optional item M1024 Payment Diagnoses (Columns 3 and 4) may be completed. A case mix diagnosis is a diagnosis that determines the Medicare P P S case mix group. Do not assign symptom control ratings for V- or E-codes.

Code each row according to the following directions for each column:

Column 1:   Enter the description of the diagnosis.

Column 2:   Enter the ICD-9-C M code for the diagnosis described in Column 1;

Rate the degree of symptom control for the condition listed in Column 1 using the following scale:

0 - Asymptomatic, no treatment needed at this time

1 - Symptoms well controlled with current therapy

2 - Symptoms controlled with difficulty, affecting daily functioning; patient needs ongoing monitoring

3 - Symptoms poorly controlled; patient needs frequent adjustment in treatment and dose monitoring

4 - Symptoms poorly controlled; history of re-hospitalizations

Note that in Column 2 the rating for symptom control of each diagnosis should not be used to determine the sequencing of the diagnoses listed in Column 1. These are separate items and sequencing may not coincide. Sequencing of diagnoses should reflect the seriousness of each condition and support the disciplines and services provided.

Column 3:   (OPTIONAL) If a V-code is assigned to any row in Column 2, in place of a case mix diagnosis, it may be necessary to complete optional item M1024 Payment Diagnoses (Columns 3 and 4). See OASIS-C Guidance Manual.

Column 4:   (OPTIONAL) If a V-code in Column 2 is reported in place of a case mix diagnosis that requires multiple diagnosis codes under ICD-9-C M coding guidelines, enter the diagnosis descriptions and the ICD-9-C M codes in the same row in Columns 3 and 4. For example, if the case mix diagnosis is a manifestation code, record the diagnosis description and ICD-9-C M code for the underlying condition in Column 3 of that row and the diagnosis description and ICD-9-C M code for the manifestation in Column 4 of that row. Otherwise, leave Column 4 blank in that row.

(Form on next page)

APPENDIX

OMB #0938-0760

Expiration date 7/31/2012

(M1020) Primary Diagnosis & (M1022) Other Diagnoses		(M1024) Payment Diagnoses (OPTIONAL)	
Column 1	Column 2	Column 3	Column 4
Diagnoses (Sequencing of diagnoses should reflect the seriousness of each condition and support the disciplines and services provided.)	ICD-9-C M and symptom control rating for each condition. Note that the sequencing of these ratings may not match the sequencing of the diagnoses	Complete if a V-code is assigned under certain circumstances to Column 2 in place of a case mix diagnosis.	Complete **only if** the V-code in Column 2 is reported in place of a case mix diagnosis that is a multiple coding situation (e.g., a manifestation code).
Description	ICD-9-C M / Symptom Control Rating	Description/ ICD-9-C M	Description/ ICD-9-C M
(M1020) Primary Diagnosis a. _____	**(V-codes are allowed)** a. (_ _ _ . _ _) □0 □1 □2 □3 □4	**(V- or E-codes NOT allowed)** a._____ (_ _ _ . _ _)	**(V- or E-codes NOT allowed)** a._____ (_ _ _ . _ _)
(M1022) Other Diagnoses b. _____	**(V- or E-codes are allowed)** b. (_ _ _ _ . _ _) □0 □1 □2 □3 □4	**(V- or E-codes NOT allowed)** b._____ (_ _ _ . _ _)	**(V- or E-codes NOT allowed)** b._____ (_ _ _ . _ _)
c. _____	c. (_ _ _ _ . _ _) □0 □1 □2 □3 □4	c._____ (_ _ _ . _ _)	c._____ (_ _ _ . _ _)
d. _____	d. (_ _ _ _ . _ _) □0 □1 □2 □3 □4	d._____ (_ _ _ . _ _)	d._____ (_ _ _ . _ _)
e. _____	e. (_ _ _ _ . _ _) □0 □1 □2 □3 □4	e._____ (_ _ _ . _ _)	e._____ (_ _ _ . _ _)
f. _____	f. (_ _ _ _ . _ _) □0 □1 □2 □3 □4	f._____ (_ _ _ . _ _)	f._____ (_ _ _ . _ _)

(M1030) Therapies the patient receives <u>at home</u>: **(Mark all that apply.)**

- ☐ 1 - Intravenous or infusion therapy (excludes TPN)
- ☐ 2 - Parenteral nutrition (TPN or lipids)
- ☐ 3 - Enteral nutrition (nasogastric, gastrostomy, jejunostomy, or any other artificial entry into the alimentary canal)
- ☐ 4 - None of the above

(M1032) Risk for Hospitalization: Which of the following signs or symptoms characterize this patient as at risk for hospitalization? **(Mark all that apply.)**

- ☐ 1 - Recent decline in mental, emotional, or behavioral status
- ☐ 2 - Multiple hospitalizations (2 or more) in the past 12 months
- ☐ 3 - History of falls (2 or more falls - or any fall with an injury - in the past year)
- ☐ 4 - Taking five or more medications
- ☐ 5 - Frailty indicators, e.g., weight loss, self-reported exhaustion
- ☐ 6 - Other
- ☐ 7 - None of the above

 181

APPENDIX

OMB #0938-0760   Expiration date 7/31/2012

(M1034) Overall Status: Which description best fits the patient's overall status? **(Check one)**

☐ 0 - The patient is stable with no heightened risk(s) for serious complications and death (beyond those typical of the patient's age).

☐ 1 - The patient is temporarily facing high health risk(s) but is likely to return to being stable without heightened risk(s) for serious complications and death (beyond those typical of the patient's age).

☐ 2 - The patient is likely to remain in fragile health and have ongoing high risk(s) of serious complications and death.

☐ 3 - The patient has serious progressive conditions that could lead to death within a year.

☐ UK - The patient's situation is unknown or unclear.

(M1036) Risk Factors, either present or past, likely to affect current health status and/or outcome: **(Mark all that apply.)**

☐ 1 - Smoking

☐ 2 - Obesity

☐ 3 - Alcohol dependency

☐ 4 - Drug dependency

☐ 5 - None of the above

☐ UK - Unknown

(M1040) Influenza Vaccine: Did the patient receive the influenza vaccine from your agency for this year's influenza season (October 1 through March 31) during this episode of care?

☐ 0 - No

☐ 1 - Yes [*Go to M1050*]

☐ NA - Does not apply because entire episode of care (SOC/ROC to Transfer/Discharge) is outside this influenza season. [*Go to M1050*]

(M1045) Reason Influenza Vaccine not received: If the patient did not receive the influenza vaccine from your agency during this episode of care, state reason:

☐ 1 - Received from another health care provider (e.g., physician)

☐ 2 - Received from your agency previously during this year's flu season

☐ 3 - Offered and declined

☐ 4 - Assessed and determined to have medical contraindication(s)

☐ 5 - Not indicated; patient does not meet age/condition guidelines for influenza vaccine

☐ 6 - Inability to obtain vaccine due to declared shortage

☐ 7 - None of the above

(M1050) Pneumococcal Vaccine: Did the patient receive pneumococcal polysaccharide vaccine (PPV) from your agency during this episode of care (SOC/ROC to Transfer/Discharge)?

☐ 0 - No

☐ 1 - Yes [*Go to M1500 at TRN; Go to M1230 at DC*]

(M1055) Reason PPV not received: If patient did not receive the pneumococcal polysaccharide vaccine (PPV) from your agency during this episode of care (SOC/ROC to Transfer/Discharge), state reason:

☐ 1 - Patient has received PPV in the past

☐ 2 - Offered and declined

☐ 3 - Assessed and determined to have medical contraindication(s)

☐ 4 - Not indicated; patient does not meet age/condition guidelines for PPV

☐ 5 - None of the above

APPENDIX

OMB #0938-0760

Expiration date 7/31/2012

LIVING ARRANGEMENTS

(M1100) **Patient Living Situation:** Which of the following best describes the patient's residential circumstance and availability of assistance? **(Check one box only.)**

Living Arrangement	Availability of Assistance				
	Around the clock	Regular daytime	Regular nighttime	Occasional / short-term assistance	No assistance available
a. Patient lives alone	☐ 01	☐ 02	☐ 03	☐ 04	☐ 05
b. Patient lives with other person(s) in the home	☐ 06	☐ 07	☐ 08	☐ 09	☐ 10
c. Patient lives in congregate situation (e.g., assisted living)	☐ 11	☐ 12	☐ 13	☐ 14	☐ 15

SENSORY STATUS

(M1200) **Vision** (with corrective lenses if the patient usually wears them):

- ☐ 0 - Normal vision: sees adequately in most situations; can see medication labels, newsprint.
- ☐ 1 - Partially impaired: cannot see medication labels or newsprint, but <u>can</u> see obstacles in path, and the surrounding layout; can count fingers at arm's length.
- ☐ 2 - Severely impaired: cannot locate objects without hearing or touching them or patient nonresponsive.

(M1210) **Ability to hear** (with hearing aid or hearing appliance if normally used):

- ☐ 0 - Adequate: hears normal conversation without difficulty.
- ☐ 1 - Mildly to Moderately Impaired: difficulty hearing in some environments or speaker may need to increase volume or speak distinctly.
- ☐ 2 - Severely Impaired: absence of useful hearing.
- ☐ UK - Unable to assess hearing.

(M1220) **Understanding of Verbal Content** in patient's own language (with hearing aid or device if used):

- ☐ 0 - Understands: clear comprehension without cues or repetitions.
- ☐ 1 - Usually Understands: understands most conversations, but misses some part/intent of message. Requires cues at times to understand.
- ☐ 2 - Sometimes Understands: understands only basic conversations or simple, direct phrases. Frequently requires cues to understand.
- ☐ 3 - Rarely/Never Understands
- ☐ UK - Unable to assess understanding.

(M1230) **Speech and Oral (Verbal) Expression of Language (in patient's own language):**

- ☐ 0 - Expresses complex ideas, feelings, and needs clearly, completely, and easily in all situations with no observable impairment.
- ☐ 1 - Minimal difficulty in expressing ideas and needs (may take extra time; makes occasional errors in word choice, grammar or speech intelligibility; needs minimal prompting or assistance).
- ☐ 2 - Expresses simple ideas or needs with moderate difficulty (needs prompting or assistance, errors in word choice, organization or speech intelligibility). Speaks in phrases or short sentences.
- ☐ 3 - Has severe difficulty expressing basic ideas or needs and requires maximal assistance or guessing by listener. Speech limited to single words or short phrases.
- ☐ 4 - <u>Unable</u> to express basic needs even with maximal prompting or assistance but is not comatose or unresponsive (e.g., speech is nonsensical or unintelligible).
- ☐ 5 - Patient nonresponsive or unable to speak.

OMB #0938-0760   Expiration date 7/31/2012

(M1240) Has this patient had a formal **Pain Assessment** using a standardized pain assessment tool (appropriate to the patient's ability to communicate the severity of pain)?

- ☐ 0 - No standardized assessment conducted
- ☐ 1 - Yes, and it does not indicate severe pain
- ☐ 2 - Yes, and it indicates severe pain

(M1242) **Frequency of Pain Interfering** with patient's activity or movement:

- ☐ 0 - Patient has no pain
- ☐ 1 - Patient has pain that does not interfere with activity or movement
- ☐ 2 - Less often than daily
- ☐ 3 - Daily, but not constantly
- ☐ 4 - All of the time

INTEGUMENTARY STATUS

(M1300) Pressure Ulcer Assessment: Was this patient assessed for **Risk of Developing Pressure Ulcers**?

- ☐ 0 - No assessment conducted [*Go to M1306*]
- ☐ 1 - Yes, based on an evaluation of clinical factors, e.g., mobility, incontinence, nutrition, etc., without use of standardized tool
- ☐ 2 - Yes, using a standardized tool, e.g., Braden, Norton, other

(M1302) Does this patient have a **Risk of Developing Pressure Ulcers**?

- ☐ 0 - No
- ☐ 1 - Yes

(M1306) Does this patient have at least one **Unhealed Pressure Ulcer at Stage II or Higher** or designated as "unstageable"?

- ☐ 0 - No [*Go to M1322*]
- ☐ 1 - Yes

(M1307) The **Oldest Non-epithelialized Stage II Pressure Ulcer** that is present at discharge

- ☐ 1 - Was present at the most recent SOC/ROC assessment

- ☐ 2 - Developed since the most recent SOC/ROC assessment: record date pressure ulcer first identified:

    __ __ / __ __ / ____ __ __
    month / day / year

- ☐ NA - No non-epithelialized Stage II pressure ulcers are present at discharge

          The How-to Guide to Home Health Therapy Documentation

APPENDIX

OMB #0938-0760

Expiration date 7/31/2012

(M1308) Current Number of Unhealed (non-epithelialized) Pressure Ulcers at Each Stage:
(Enter "0" if none; excludes Stage I pressure ulcers)

Stage description – unhealed pressure ulcers	Column 1 Complete at SOC/ROC/FU & D/C Number Currently Present	Column 2 Complete at FU & D/C Number of those listed in Column 1 that were present on admission (most recent SOC / ROC)
a. **Stage II:** Partial thickness loss of dermis presenting as a shallow open ulcer with red pink wound bed, without slough. May also present as an intact or open/ruptured serum-filled blister.	____	____
b. **Stage III:** Full thickness tissue loss. Subcutaneous fat may be visible but bone, tendon, or muscles are not exposed. Slough may be present but does not obscure the depth of tissue loss. May include undermining and tunneling.	____	____
c. **Stage IV:** Full thickness tissue loss with visible bone, tendon, or muscle. Slough or eschar may be present on some parts of the wound bed. Often includes undermining and tunneling.	____	____
d.1 Unstageable: Known or likely but unstageable due to non-removable dressing or device	____	____
d.2 Unstageable: Known or likely but unstageable due to coverage of wound bed by slough and/or eschar.	____	____
d.3 Unstageable: Suspected deep tissue injury in evolution.	____	____

Directions for M1310, M1312, and M1314: If the patient has one or more unhealed (non-epithelialized) Stage III or IV pressure ulcers, identify the **Stage III or IV pressure ulcer with the largest surface dimension (length x width)** and record in centimeters. If no Stage III or Stage IV pressure ulcers, go to M1320.

(M1310) Pressure Ulcer Length: Longest length "head-to-toe" | ___ | ___ | . | ___ | (cm)

(M1312) Pressure Ulcer Width: Width of the same pressure ulcer; greatest width perpendicular to the length

| ___ | ___ | . | ___ | (cm)

(M1314) Pressure Ulcer Depth: Depth of the same pressure ulcer; from visible surface to the deepest area

| ___ | ___ | . | ___ | (cm)

(M1320) Status of Most Problematic (Observable) Pressure Ulcer:

☐   0 -   Newly epithelialized
☐   1 -   Fully granulating
☐   2 -   Early/partial granulation
☐   3 -   Not healing
☐ NA -   No observable pressure ulcer

APPENDIX

OMB #0938-0760

Expiration date 7/31/2012

(M1322) Current Number of Stage I Pressure Ulcers: Intact skin with non-blanchable redness of a localized area usually over a bony prominence. The area may be painful, firm, soft, warmer or cooler as compared to adjacent tissue.

☐ 0   ☐ 1   ☐ 2   ☐ 3   ☐ 4 or more

(M1324) Stage of Most Problematic Unhealed (Observable) Pressure Ulcer:

☐ 1 - Stage I
☐ 2 - Stage II
☐ 3 - Stage III
☐ 4 - Stage IV
☐ NA - No observable pressure ulcer or unhealed pressure ulcer

(M1330) Does this patient have a **Stasis Ulcer?**

☐ 0 - No [*Go to M1340*]
☐ 1 - Yes, patient has BOTH observable and unobservable stasis ulcers
☐ 2 - Yes, patient has observable stasis ulcers ONLY
☐ 3 - Yes, patient has unobservable stasis ulcers ONLY (known but not observable due to non-removable dressing) [*Go to M1340*]

(M1332) Current Number of (Observable) Stasis Ulcer(s):

☐ 1 - One
☐ 2 - Two
☐ 3 - Three
☐ 4 - Four or more

(M1334) Status of Most Problematic (Observable) Stasis Ulcer:

☐ 0 - Newly epithelialized
☐ 1 - Fully granulating
☐ 2 - Early/partial granulation
☐ 3 - Not healing

(M1340) Does this patient have a **Surgical Wound?**

☐ 0 - No [*Go to M1350*]
☐ 1 - Yes, patient has at least one (observable) surgical wound
☐ 2 - Surgical wound known but not observable due to non-removable dressing [*Go to M1350*]

(M1342) Status of Most Problematic (Observable) Surgical Wound:

☐ 0 - Newly epithelialized
☐ 1 - Fully granulating
☐ 2 - Early/partial granulation
☐ 3 - Not healing

(M1350) Does this patient have a **Skin Lesion** or **Open Wound**, excluding bowel ostomy, other than those described above that is receiving intervention by the home health agency?

☐ 0 - No
☐ 1 - Yes

APPENDIX

OMB #0938-0760

Expiration date 7/31/2012

RESPIRATORY STATUS

(M1400) When is the patient dyspneic or noticeably **Short of Breath**?

- ☐ 0 - Patient is not short of breath
- ☐ 1 - When walking more than 20 feet, climbing stairs
- ☐ 2 - With moderate exertion (e.g., while dressing, using commode or bedpan, walking distances less than 20 feet)
- ☐ 3 - With minimal exertion (e.g., while eating, talking, or performing other ADLs) or with agitation
- ☐ 4 - At rest (during day or night)

(M1410) **Respiratory Treatments** utilized at home: **(Mark all that apply.)**

- ☐ 1 - Oxygen (intermittent or continuous)
- ☐ 2 - Ventilator (continually or at night)
- ☐ 3 - Continuous / Bi-level positive airway pressure
- ☐ 4 - None of the above

CARDIAC STATUS

(M1500) **Symptoms in Heart Failure Patients:** If patient has been diagnosed with heart failure, did the patient exhibit symptoms indicated by clinical heart failure guidelines (including dyspnea, orthopnea, edema, or weight gain) at any point since the previous OASIS assessment?

- ☐ 0 - No [*Go to M2004 at TRN; Go to M1600 at DC*]
- ☐ 1 - Yes
- ☐ 2 - Not assessed [*Go to M2004 at TRN; Go to M1600 at DC*]
- ☐ NA - Patient does not have diagnosis of heart failure [*Go to M2004 at TRN; Go to M1600 at DC*]

(M1510) **Heart Failure Follow-up:** If patient has been diagnosed with heart failure and has exhibited symptoms indicative of heart failure since the previous OASIS assessment, what action(s) has (have) been taken to respond? **(Mark all that apply.)**

- ☐ 0 - No action taken
- ☐ 1 - Patient's physician (or other primary care practitioner) contacted the same day
- ☐ 2 - Patient advised to get emergency treatment (e.g., call 911 or go to emergency room)
- ☐ 3 - Implemented physician-ordered patient-specific established parameters for treatment
- ☐ 4 - Patient education or other clinical interventions
- ☐ 5 - Obtained change in care plan orders (e.g., increased monitoring by agency, change in visit frequency, telehealth, etc.)

ELIMINATION STATUS

(M1600) Has this patient been treated for a **Urinary Tract Infection** in the past 14 days?

- ☐ 0 - No
- ☐ 1 - Yes
- ☐ NA - Patient on prophylactic treatment
- ☐ UK - Unknown **[Omit "UK" option on DC]**

(M1610) **Urinary Incontinence or Urinary Catheter Presence:**

- ☐ 0 - No incontinence or catheter (includes anuria or ostomy for urinary drainage) [*Go to M1620*]
- ☐ 1 - Patient is incontinent
- ☐ 2 - Patient requires a urinary catheter (i.e., external, indwelling, intermittent, suprapubic) [*Go to M1620*]

OASIS-C: All Items
Centers for Medicare & Medicaid Services   August 2009   Page 13 of 24

OMB #0938-0760

Expiration date 7/31/2012

(M1615) When does **Urinary Incontinence** occur?

- ☐ 0 - Timed-voiding defers incontinence
- ☐ 1 - Occasional stress incontinence
- ☐ 2 - During the night only
- ☐ 3 - During the day only
- ☐ 4 - During the day and night

(M1620) Bowel Incontinence Frequency:

- ☐ 0 - Very rarely or never has bowel incontinence
- ☐ 1 - Less than once weekly
- ☐ 2 - One to three times weekly
- ☐ 3 - Four to six times weekly
- ☐ 4 - On a daily basis
- ☐ 5 - More often than once daily
- ☐ NA - Patient has ostomy for bowel elimination
- ☐ UK - Unknown **[Omit "UK" option on FU, DC]**

(M1630) Ostomy for Bowel Elimination: Does this patient have an ostomy for bowel elimination that (within the last 14 days): a) was related to an inpatient facility stay, <u>or</u> b) necessitated a change in medical or treatment regimen?

- ☐ 0 - Patient does <u>not</u> have an ostomy for bowel elimination.
- ☐ 1 - Patient's ostomy was <u>not</u> related to an inpatient stay and did <u>not</u> necessitate change in medical or treatment regimen.
- ☐ 2 - The ostomy <u>was</u> related to an inpatient stay or <u>did</u> necessitate change in medical or treatment regimen.

NEURO/EMOTIONAL/BEHAVIORAL STATUS

(M1700) Cognitive Functioning: Patient's current (day of assessment) level of alertness, orientation, comprehension, concentration, and immediate memory for simple commands.

- ☐ 0 - Alert/oriented, able to focus and shift attention, comprehends and recalls task directions independently.
- ☐ 1 - Requires prompting (cuing, repetition, reminders) only under stressful or unfamiliar conditions.
- ☐ 2 - Requires assistance and some direction in specific situations (e.g., on all tasks involving shifting of attention), or consistently requires low stimulus environment due to distractibility.
- ☐ 3 - Requires considerable assistance in routine situations. Is not alert and oriented or is unable to shift attention and recall directions more than half the time.
- ☐ 4 - Totally dependent due to disturbances such as constant disorientation, coma, persistent vegetative state, or delirium.

(M1710) When Confused (Reported or Observed Within the Last 14 Days):

- ☐ 0 - Never
- ☐ 1 - In new or complex situations only
- ☐ 2 - On awakening or at night only
- ☐ 3 - During the day and evening, but not constantly
- ☐ 4 - Constantly
- ☐ NA - Patient nonresponsive

APPENDIX

OMB #0938-0760

Expiration date 7/31/2012

(M1720) **When Anxious (Reported or Observed Within the Last 14 Days):**

☐ 0 - None of the time

☐ 1 - Less often than daily

☐ 2 - Daily, but not constantly

☐ 3 - All of the time

☐ NA - Patient nonresponsive

(M1730) **Depression Screening:** Has the patient been screened for depression, using a standardized depression screening tool?

☐ 0 - No

☐ 1 - Yes, patient was screened using the PHQ-2©* scale. (Instructions for this two-question tool: Ask patient: "Over the last two weeks, how often have you been bothered by any of the following problems")

PHQ-2©*	Not at all 0 - 1 day	Several days 2 - 6 days	More than half of the days 7 – 11 days	Nearly every day 12 – 14 days	N/A Unable to respond
a) Little interest or pleasure in doing things	☐0	☐1	☐2	☐3	☐na
b) Feeling down, depressed, or hopeless?	☐0	☐1	☐2	☐3	☐na

☐ 2 - Yes, with a different standardized assessment-and the patient meets criteria for further evaluation for depression.

☐ 3 - Yes, patient was screened with a different standardized assessment-and the patient does not meet criteria for further evaluation for depression.

Copyright© Pfizer Inc. All rights reserved. Reproduced with permission.

(M1740) **Cognitive, behavioral, and psychiatric symptoms** that are demonstrated <u>at least once a week</u> (Reported or Observed): **(Mark all that apply.)**

☐ 1 - Memory deficit: failure to recognize familiar persons/places, inability to recall events of past 24 hours, significant memory loss so that supervision is required

☐ 2 - Impaired decision-making: failure to perform usual ADLs or IADLs, inability to appropriately stop activities, jeopardizes safety through actions

☐ 3 - Verbal disruption: yelling, threatening, excessive profanity, sexual references, etc.

☐ 4 - Physical aggression: aggressive or combative to self and others (e.g., hits self, throws objects, punches, dangerous maneuvers with wheelchair or other objects)

☐ 5 - Disruptive, infantile, or socially inappropriate behavior (**excludes** verbal actions)

☐ 6 - Delusional, hallucinatory, or paranoid behavior

☐ 7 - None of the above behaviors demonstrated

(M1745) **Frequency of Disruptive Behavior Symptoms (Reported or Observed)** Any physical, verbal, or other disruptive/dangerous symptoms that are injurious to self or others or jeopardize personal safety.

☐ 0 - Never

☐ 1 - Less than once a month

☐ 2 - Once a month

☐ 3 - Several times each month

☐ 4 - Several times a week

☐ 5 - At least daily

OASIS-C: All Items
Centers for Medicare & Medicaid Services   August 2009   Page 15 of 24

APPENDIX

OMB #0938-0760

Expiration date 7/31/2012

(M1750) Is this patient receiving **Psychiatric Nursing Services** at home provided by a qualified psychiatric nurse?

- ☐ 0 - No
- ☐ 1 - Yes

ADL/IADLs

(M1800) Grooming: Current ability to tend safely to personal hygiene needs (i.e., washing face and hands, hair care, shaving or make up, teeth or denture care, fingernail care).

- ☐ 0 - Able to groom self unaided, with or without the use of assistive devices or adapted methods.
- ☐ 1 - Grooming utensils must be placed within reach before able to complete grooming activities.
- ☐ 2 - Someone must assist the patient to groom self.
- ☐ 3 - Patient depends entirely upon someone else for grooming needs.

(M1810) Current **Ability to Dress Upper Body** safely (with or without dressing aids) including undergarments, pullovers, front-opening shirts and blouses, managing zippers, buttons, and snaps:

- ☐ 0 - Able to get clothes out of closets and drawers, put them on and remove them from the upper body without assistance.
- ☐ 1 - Able to dress upper body without assistance if clothing is laid out or handed to the patient.
- ☐ 2 - Someone must help the patient put on upper body clothing.
- ☐ 3 - Patient depends entirely upon another person to dress the upper body.

(M1820) Current **Ability to Dress Lower Body** safely (with or without dressing aids) including undergarments, slacks, socks or nylons, shoes:

- ☐ 0 - Able to obtain, put on, and remove clothing and shoes without assistance.
- ☐ 1 - Able to dress lower body without assistance if clothing and shoes are laid out or handed to the patient.
- ☐ 2 - Someone must help the patient put on undergarments, slacks, socks or nylons, and shoes.
- ☐ 3 - Patient depends entirely upon another person to dress lower body.

(M1830) Bathing: Current ability to wash entire body safely. **Excludes grooming (washing face, washing hands, and shampooing hair).**

- ☐ 0 - Able to bathe self in shower or tub independently, including getting in and out of tub/shower.
- ☐ 1 - With the use of devices, is able to bathe self in shower or tub independently, including getting in and out of the tub/shower.
- ☐ 2 - Able to bathe in shower or tub with the intermittent assistance of another person:
  - (a) for intermittent supervision or encouragement or reminders, OR
  - (b) to get in and out of the shower or tub, OR
  - (c) for washing difficult to reach areas.
- ☐ 3 - Able to participate in bathing self in shower or tub, but requires presence of another person throughout the bath for assistance or supervision.
- ☐ 4 - Unable to use the shower or tub, but able to bathe self independently with or without the use of devices at the sink, in chair, or on commode.
- ☐ 5 - Unable to use the shower or tub, but able to participate in bathing self in bed, at the sink, in bedside chair, or on commode, with the assistance or supervision of another person throughout the bath.
- ☐ 6 - Unable to participate effectively in bathing and is bathed totally by another person.

APPENDIX

OMB #0938-0760   Expiration date 7/31/2012

(M1840) Toilet Transferring: Current ability to get to and from the toilet or bedside commode safely <u>and</u> transfer on and off toilet/commode.

- ☐ 0 - Able to get to and from the toilet and transfer independently with or without a device.
- ☐ 1 - When reminded, assisted, or supervised by another person, able to get to and from the toilet and transfer.
- ☐ 2 - <u>Unable</u> to get to and from the toilet but is able to use a bedside commode (with or without assistance).
- ☐ 3 - <u>Unable</u> to get to and from the toilet or bedside commode but is able to use a bedpan/urinal independently.
- ☐ 4 - Is totally dependent in toileting.

(M1845) Toileting Hygiene: Current ability to maintain perineal hygiene safely, adjust clothes and/or incontinence pads before and after using toilet, commode, bedpan, urinal. If managing ostomy, includes cleaning area around stoma, but not managing equipment.

- ☐ 0 - Able to manage toileting hygiene and clothing management without assistance.
- ☐ 1 - Able to manage toileting hygiene and clothing management without assistance if supplies/implements are laid out for the patient.
- ☐ 2 - Someone must help the patient to maintain toileting hygiene and/or adjust clothing.
- ☐ 3 - Patient depends entirely upon another person to maintain toileting hygiene.

(M1850) Transferring: Current ability to move safely from bed to chair, or ability to turn and position self in bed if patient is bedfast.

- ☐ 0 - Able to independently transfer.
- ☐ 1 - Able to transfer with minimal human assistance or with use of an assistive device.
- ☐ 2 - Able to bear weight and pivot during the transfer process but unable to transfer self.
- ☐ 3 - Unable to transfer self and is unable to bear weight or pivot when transferred by another person.
- ☐ 4 - Bedfast, unable to transfer but is able to turn and position self in bed.
- ☐ 5 - Bedfast, unable to transfer and is unable to turn and position self.

(M1860) Ambulation/Locomotion: Current ability to walk safely, once in a standing position, or use a wheelchair, once in a seated position, on a variety of surfaces.

- ☐ 0 - Able to independently walk on even and uneven surfaces and negotiate stairs with or without railings (i.e., needs no human assistance or assistive device).
- ☐ 1 - With the use of a one-handed device (e.g. cane, single crutch, hemi-walker), able to independently walk on even and uneven surfaces and negotiate stairs with or without railings.
- ☐ 2 - Requires use of a two-handed device (e.g., walker or crutches) to walk alone on a level surface and/or requires human supervision or assistance to negotiate stairs or steps or uneven surfaces.
- ☐ 3 - Able to walk only with the supervision or assistance of another person at all times.
- ☐ 4 - Chairfast, <u>unable</u> to ambulate but is able to wheel self independently.
- ☐ 5 - Chairfast, unable to ambulate and is <u>unable</u> to wheel self.
- ☐ 6 - Bedfast, unable to ambulate or be up in a chair.

(M1870) Feeding or Eating: Current ability to feed self meals and snacks safely. Note: This refers only to the process of <u>eating</u>, <u>chewing</u>, and <u>swallowing</u>, <u>not preparing</u> the food to be eaten.

- ☐ 0 - Able to independently feed self.
- ☐ 1 - Able to feed self independently but requires:
    - (a) meal set-up; <u>OR</u>
    - (b) intermittent assistance or supervision from another person; <u>OR</u>
    - (c) a liquid, pureed or ground meat diet.
- ☐ 2 - <u>Unable</u> to feed self and must be assisted or supervised throughout the meal/snack.
- ☐ 3 - Able to take in nutrients orally <u>and</u> receives supplemental nutrients through a nasogastric tube or gastrostomy.
- ☐ 4 - <u>Unable</u> to take in nutrients orally and is fed nutrients through a nasogastric tube or gastrostomy.
- ☐ 5 - Unable to take in nutrients orally or by tube feeding.

OASIS-C: All Items
Centers for Medicare & Medicaid Services   August 2009   Page 17 of 24

APPENDIX

OMB #0938-0760

Expiration date 7/31/2012

(M1880) Current **Ability to Plan and Prepare Light Meals** (e.g., cereal, sandwich) or reheat delivered meals safely:

- ☐ 0 - (a) Able to independently plan and prepare all light meals for self or reheat delivered meals; <u>OR</u>
  (b) Is physically, cognitively, and mentally able to prepare light meals on a regular basis but has not routinely performed light meal preparation in the past (i.e., prior to this home care admission).
- ☐ 1 - <u>Unable</u> to prepare light meals on a regular basis due to physical, cognitive, or mental limitations.
- ☐ 2 - Unable to prepare any light meals or reheat any delivered meals.

(M1890) Ability to Use Telephone: Current ability to answer the phone safely, including dialing numbers, and <u>effectively</u> using the telephone to communicate.

- ☐ 0 - Able to dial numbers and answer calls appropriately and as desired.
- ☐ 1 - Able to use a specially adapted telephone (i.e., large numbers on the dial, teletype phone for the deaf) and call essential numbers.
- ☐ 2 - Able to answer the telephone and carry on a normal conversation but has difficulty with placing calls.
- ☐ 3 - Able to answer the telephone only some of the time or is able to carry on only a limited conversation.
- ☐ 4 - <u>Unable</u> to answer the telephone at all but can listen if assisted with equipment.
- ☐ 5 - Totally unable to use the telephone.
- ☐ NA - Patient does not have a telephone.

(M1900) Prior Functioning ADL/IADL: Indicate the patient's usual ability with everyday activities prior to this current illness, exacerbation, or injury. Check only **one** box in each row.

Functional Area	Independent	Needed Some Help	Dependent
a. Self-Care (e.g., grooming, dressing, and bathing)	☐0	☐1	☐2
b. Ambulation	☐0	☐1	☐2
c. Transfer	☐0	☐1	☐2
d. Household tasks (e.g., light meal preparation, laundry, shopping)	☐0	☐1	☐2

(M1910) Has this patient had a multi-factor **Fall Risk Assessment** (such as falls history, use of multiple medications, mental impairment, toileting frequency, general mobility/transferring impairment, environmental hazards)?

- ☐ 0 - No multi-factor falls risk assessment conducted.
- ☐ 1 - Yes, and it does not indicate a risk for falls.
- ☐ 2 - Yes, and it indicates a risk for falls.

MEDICATIONS

(M2000) Drug Regimen Review: Does a complete drug regimen review indicate potential clinically significant medication issues, e.g., drug reactions, ineffective drug therapy, side effects, drug interactions, duplicate therapy, omissions, dosage errors, or noncompliance?

- ☐ 0 - Not assessed/reviewed **[*Go to M2010*]**
- ☐ 1 - No problems found during review **[*Go to M2010*]**
- ☐ 2 - Problems found during review
- ☐ NA - Patient is not taking any medications **[*Go to M2040*]**

(M2002) Medication Follow-up: Was a physician or the physician-designee contacted within one calendar day to resolve clinically significant medication issues, including reconciliation?

- ☐ 0 - No
- ☐ 1 - Yes

OASIS-C: All Items
Centers for Medicare & Medicaid Services   August 2009   Page 18 of 24

APPENDIX

OMB #0938-0760

Expiration date 7/31/2012

(M2004) Medication Intervention: If there were any clinically significant medication issues since the previous OASIS assessment, was a physician or the physician-designee contacted within one calendar day of the assessment to resolve clinically significant medication issues, including reconciliation?

☐ 0 - No

☐ 1 - Yes

☐ NA - No clinically significant medication issues identified since the previous OASIS assessment

(M2010) Patient/Caregiver High Risk Drug Education: Has the patient/caregiver received instruction on special precautions for all high-risk medications (such as hypoglycemics, anticoagulants, etc.) and how and when to report problems that may occur?

☐ 0 - No

☐ 1 - Yes

☐ NA - Patient not taking any high risk drugs OR patient/caregiver fully knowledgeable about special precautions associated with all high-risk medications

(M2015) Patient/Caregiver Drug Education Intervention: Since the previous OASIS assessment, was the patient/caregiver instructed by agency staff or other health care provider to monitor the effectiveness of drug therapy, drug reactions, and side effects, and how and when to report problems that may occur?

☐ 0 - No

☐ 1 - Yes

☐ NA - Patient not taking any drugs

(M2020) Management of Oral Medications: Patient's current ability to prepare and take all oral medications reliably and safely, including administration of the correct dosage at the appropriate times/intervals. **Excludes injectable and IV medications. (NOTE: This refers to ability, not compliance or willingness.)**

☐ 0 - Able to independently take the correct oral medication(s) and proper dosage(s) at the correct times.

☐ 1 - Able to take medication(s) at the correct times if:
(a) individual dosages are prepared in advance by another person; OR
(b) another person develops a drug diary or chart.

☐ 2 - Able to take medication(s) at the correct times if given reminders by another person at the appropriate times

☐ 3 - Unable to take medication unless administered by another person.

☐ NA - No oral medications prescribed.

(M2030) Management of Injectable Medications: Patient's current ability to prepare and take all prescribed injectable medications reliably and safely, including administration of correct dosage at the appropriate times/intervals. **Excludes IV medications.**

☐ 0 - Able to independently take the correct medication(s) and proper dosage(s) at the correct times.

☐ 1 - Able to take injectable medication(s) at the correct times if:
(a) individual syringes are prepared in advance by another person; OR
(b) another person develops a drug diary or chart.

☐ 2 - Able to take medication(s) at the correct times if given reminders by another person based on the frequency of the injection

☐ 3 - Unable to take injectable medication unless administered by another person.

☐ NA - No injectable medications prescribed.

(M2040) Prior Medication Management: Indicate the patient's usual ability with managing oral and injectable medications prior to this current illness, exacerbation, or injury. Check only **one** box in each row.

Functional Area	Independent	Needed Some Help	Dependent	Not Applicable
a. Oral medications	☐0	☐1	☐2	☐na
b. Injectable medications	☐0	☐1	☐2	☐na

APPENDIX

OMB #0938-0760

Expiration date 7/31/2012

CARE MANAGEMENT

(M2100) Types and Sources of Assistance: Determine the level of caregiver ability and willingness to provide assistance for the following activities, if assistance is needed. (Check only **one** box in each row.)

Type of Assistance	No assistance needed in this area	Caregiver(s) currently provide assistance	Caregiver(s) need training/ supportive services to provide assistance	Caregiver(s) not likely to provide assistance	Unclear if Caregiver(s) will provide assistance	Assistance needed, but no Caregiver(s) available
a. **ADL assistance** (e.g., transfer/ ambulation, bathing, dressing, toileting, eating/feeding)	☐0	☐1	☐2	☐3	☐4	☐5
b. **IADL assistance** (e.g., meals, housekeeping, laundry, telephone, shopping, finances)	☐0	☐1	☐2	☐3	☐4	☐5
c. **Medication administration** (e.g., oral, inhaled or injectable)	☐0	☐1	☐2	☐3	☐4	☐5
d. **Medical procedures/ treatments** (e.g., changing wound dressing)	☐0	☐1	☐2	☐3	☐4	☐5
e. **Management of Equipment** (includes oxygen, IV/infusion equipment, enteral/ parenteral nutrition, ventilator therapy equipment or supplies)	☐0	☐1	☐2	☐3	☐4	☐5
f. **Supervision and safety** (e.g., due to cognitive impairment)	☐0	☐1	☐2	☐3	☐4	☐5
g. **Advocacy or facilitation** of patient's participation in appropriate medical care (includes transporta-tion to or from appointments)	☐0	☐1	☐2	☐3	☐4	☐5

OASIS-C: All Items
Centers for Medicare & Medicaid Services   August 2009   Page 20 of 24

APPENDIX

OMB #0938-0760

Expiration date 7/31/2012

(M2110) **How Often** does the patient receive **ADL or IADL assistance** from any caregiver(s) (other than home health agency staff)?

- ☐ 1 - At least daily
- ☐ 2 - Three or more times per week
- ☐ 3 - One to two times per week
- ☐ 4 - Received, but less often than weekly
- ☐ 5 - No assistance received
- ☐ UK - Unknown **[Omit "UK" option on DC]**

THERAPY NEED AND PLAN OF CARE

(M2200) **Therapy Need:** In the home health plan of care for the Medicare payment episode for which this assessment will define a case mix group, what is the indicated need for therapy visits (total of reasonable and necessary physical, occupational, and speech-language pathology visits combined)? **(Enter zero ["000"] if no therapy visits indicated.)**

(__ __ __) Number of therapy visits indicated (total of physical, occupational and speech-language pathology combined).

- ☐ NA - Not Applicable: No case mix group defined by this assessment.

(M2250) **Plan of Care Synopsis:** (Check only **one** box in each row.) Does the physician-ordered plan of care include the following:

Plan / Intervention	No	Yes	Not Applicable	
a. Patient-specific parameters for notifying physician of changes in vital signs or other clinical findings	☐0	☐1	☐na	Physician has chosen not to establish patient-specific parameters for this patient. Agency will use standardized clinical guidelines accessible for all care providers to reference
b. Diabetic foot care including monitoring for the presence of skin lesions on the lower extremities and patient/caregiver education on proper foot care	☐0	☐1	☐na	Patient is not diabetic or is bilateral amputee
c. Falls prevention interventions	☐0	☐1	☐na	Patient is not assessed to be at risk for falls
d. Depression intervention(s) such as medication, referral for other treatment, or a monitoring plan for current treatment	☐0	☐1	☐na	Patient has no diagnosis or symptoms of depression
e. Intervention(s) to monitor and mitigate pain	☐0	☐1	☐na	No pain identified
f. Intervention(s) to prevent pressure ulcers	☐0	☐1	☐na	Patient is not assessed to be at risk for pressure ulcers
g. Pressure ulcer treatment based on principles of moist wound healing OR order for treatment based on moist wound healing has been requested from physician	☐0	☐1	☐na	Patient has no pressure ulcers with need for moist wound healing

            195

APPENDIX

OMB #0938-0760

Expiration date 7/31/2012

EMERGENT CARE

(M2300) Emergent Care: Since the last time OASIS data were collected, has the patient utilized a hospital emergency department (includes holding/observation)?

- ☐ 0 - No [*Go to M2400*]
- ☐ 1 - Yes, used hospital emergency department WITHOUT hospital admission
- ☐ 2 - Yes, used hospital emergency department WITH hospital admission
- ☐ UK - Unknown [*Go to M2400*]

(M2310) Reason for Emergent Care: For what reason(s) did the patient receive emergent care (with or without hospitalization)? **(Mark all that apply.)**

- ☐ 1 - Improper medication administration, medication side effects, toxicity, anaphylaxis
- ☐ 2 - Injury caused by fall
- ☐ 3 - Respiratory infection (e.g., pneumonia, bronchitis)
- ☐ 4 - Other respiratory problem
- ☐ 5 - Heart failure (e.g., fluid overload)
- ☐ 6 - Cardiac dysrhythmia (irregular heartbeat)
- ☐ 7 - Myocardial infarction or chest pain
- ☐ 8 - Other heart disease
- ☐ 9 - Stroke (CVA) or TIA
- ☐ 10 - Hypo/Hyperglycemia, diabetes out of control
- ☐ 11 - GI bleeding, obstruction, constipation, impaction
- ☐ 12 - Dehydration, malnutrition
- ☐ 13 - Urinary tract infection
- ☐ 14 - IV catheter-related infection or complication
- ☐ 15 - Wound infection or deterioration
- ☐ 16 - Uncontrolled pain
- ☐ 17 - Acute mental/behavioral health problem
- ☐ 18 - Deep vein thrombosis, pulmonary embolus
- ☐ 19 - Other than above reasons
- ☐ UK - Reason unknown

          The How-to Guide to Home Health Therapy Documentation

APPENDIX

OMB #0938-0760 Expiration date 7/31/2012

DATA ITEMS COLLECTED AT INPATIENT FACILITY ADMISSION OR AGENCY DISCHARGE ONLY

(M2400) Intervention Synopsis: (Check only **one** box in each row.) Since the previous OASIS assessment, were the following interventions BOTH included in the physician-ordered plan of care AND implemented?

Plan / Intervention	No	Yes	Not Applicable	
a. Diabetic foot care including monitoring for the presence of skin lesions on the lower extremities and patient/caregiver education on proper foot care	☐0	☐1	☐na	Patient is not diabetic or is bilateral amputee
b. Falls prevention interventions	☐0	☐1	☐na	Formal multi-factor Fall Risk Assessment indicates the patient was not at risk for falls since the last OASIS assessment
c. Depression intervention(s) such as medication, referral for other treatment, or a monitoring plan for current treatment	☐0	☐1	☐na	Formal assessment indicates patient did not meet criteria for depression AND patient did not have diagnosis of depression since the last OASIS assessment
d. Intervention(s) to monitor and mitigate pain	☐0	☐1	☐na	Formal assessment did not indicate pain since the last OASIS assessment
e. Intervention(s) to prevent pressure ulcers	☐0	☐1	☐na	Formal assessment indicates the patient was not at risk of pressure ulcers since the last OASIS assessment
f. Pressure ulcer treatment based on principles of moist wound healing	☐0	☐1	☐na	Dressings that support the principles of moist wound healing not indicated for this patient's pressure ulcers OR patient has no pressure ulcers with need for moist wound healing

(M2410) To which **Inpatient Facility** has the patient been admitted?

- ☐ 1 - Hospital [*Go to M2430*]
- ☐ 2 - Rehabilitation facility [*Go to M0903*]
- ☐ 3 - Nursing home [*Go to M2440*]
- ☐ 4 - Hospice [*Go to M0903*]
- ☐ NA - No inpatient facility admission **[Omit "NA" option on TRN]**

(M2420) Discharge Disposition: Where is the patient after discharge from your agency? **(Choose only one answer.)**

- ☐ 1 - Patient remained in the community (without formal assistive services)
- ☐ 2 - Patient remained in the community (with formal assistive services)
- ☐ 3 - Patient transferred to a non-institutional hospice
- ☐ 4 - Unknown because patient moved to a geographic location not served by this agency
- ☐ UK - Other unknown

[*Go to M0903*]

APPENDIX

OMB #0938-0760

Expiration date 7/31/2012

(M2430) **Reason for Hospitalization**: For what reason(s) did the patient require hospitalization? **(Mark all that apply.)**

- ☐ 1 - Improper medication administration, medication side effects, toxicity, anaphylaxis
- ☐ 2 - Injury caused by fall
- ☐ 3 - Respiratory infection (e.g., pneumonia, bronchitis)
- ☐ 4 - Other respiratory problem
- ☐ 5 - Heart failure (e.g., fluid overload)
- ☐ 6 - Cardiac dysrhythmia (irregular heartbeat)
- ☐ 7 - Myocardial infarction or chest pain
- ☐ 8 - Other heart disease
- ☐ 9 - Stroke (CVA) or TIA
- ☐ 10 - Hypo/Hyperglycemia, diabetes out of control
- ☐ 11 - GI bleeding, obstruction, constipation, impaction
- ☐ 12 - Dehydration, malnutrition
- ☐ 13 - Urinary tract infection
- ☐ 14 - IV catheter-related infection or complication
- ☐ 15 - Wound infection or deterioration
- ☐ 16 - Uncontrolled pain
- ☐ 17 - Acute mental/behavioral health problem
- ☐ 18 - Deep vein thrombosis, pulmonary embolus
- ☐ 19 - Scheduled treatment or procedure
- ☐ 20 - Other than above reasons
- ☐ UK - Reason unknown

[*Go to M0903*]

(M2440) For what **Reason(s)** was the patient **Admitted** to a **Nursing Home**? **(Mark all that apply.)**

- ☐ 1 - Therapy services
- ☐ 2 - Respite care
- ☐ 3 - Hospice care
- ☐ 4 - Permanent placement
- ☐ 5 - Unsafe for care at home
- ☐ 6 - Other
- ☐ UK - Unknown

[*Go to M0903*]

(M0903) **Date of Last (Most Recent) Home Visit:**

__ __ / __ __ / __ __ __ __
month / day / year

(M0906) **Discharge/Transfer/Death Date:** Enter the date of the discharge, transfer, or death (at home) of the patient.

__ __ / __ __ / __ __ __ __
month / day / year

OASIS-C: All Items
Centers for Medicare & Medicaid Services   August 2009   Page 24 of 24

CMS Manual System	Department of Health & Human Services (DHHS)
Pub 100-02 Medicare Benefit Policy	Centers for Medicare & Medicaid Services (CMS)
Transmittal:142	Date: April 15, 2011
	Change Request 7374

SUBJECT: Home Health Therapy Services

I. SUMMARY OF CHANGES: The policy in chapter 7 is being updated due to the Calendar Year 2011 Final Rule for Home Health provisions related to therapy services provided in the home health setting and corresponding regulation text changes. Therapy provisions for this rule are effective April 1, 2011.

EFFECTIVE DATE: April 1, 2011
IMPLEMENTATION DATE: May 5, 2011

Disclaimer for manual changes only: The revision date and transmittal number apply only to red italicized material. Any other material was previously published and remains unchanged. However, if this revision contains a table of contents, you will receive the new/revised information only, and not the entire table of contents.

II. CHANGES IN MANUAL INSTRUCTIONS: (N/A if manual is not updated)
R=REVISED, N=NEW, D=DELETED

R/N/D	CHAPTER / SECTION / SUBSECTION / TITLE
R	7/40.1.2.1/Observation and Assessment of the Patient's Condition When Only the Specialized Skills of a Medical Professional Can Determine Patient's Status
R	7/40.2.1/General Principles Governing Reasonable and Necessary Physical Therapy, Speech-Language Pathology Services, and Occupational Therapy
R	7/40.2.2/Application of the Principles to Physical Therapy Services
R	7/40.2.3/Application of the General Principles to Speech-Language Pathology Services
R	7/40.2.4.1/Assessment

III. FUNDING:
For Fiscal Intermediaries (FIs), Regional Home Health Intermediaries (RHHIs) and/or Carriers:

No additional funding will be provided by CMS; contractor activities are to be carried out within their operating budgets.

For Medicare Administrative Contractors (MACs):

The Medicare Administrative Contractor is hereby advised that this constitutes technical direction as defined in your contract. CMS does not construe this as a change to the MAC Statement of Work. The contractor is not obligated to incur costs in excess of the amounts allotted in your contract unless and until specifically authorized by the contracting officer. If the contractor considers anything provided, as described above, to be outside the current scope of work, the contractor shall withhold performance on the part(s) in question and immediately notify the contracting officer, in writing or by e-mail, and request formal directions regarding continued performance requirements.

IV. ATTACHMENTS:

Business Requirements

Manual Instruction

Unless otherwise specified, the effective date is the date of service.

Attachment - Business Requirements

Pub. 100-02	Transmittal: 142	Date: April 15, 2011	Change Request: 7374

SUBJECT: Home Health Therapy Services

Effective Date: April 1, 2011
Implementation Date: May 5, 2011

I. GENERAL INFORMATION

A. Background: The policy in Pub. 100-02, Medicare Benefit Policy Manual, chapter 7, is being updated due to the Calendar Year 2011 Final Rule for Home Health provisions related to therapy services provided in the home health setting and corresponding regulation text changes. Therapy provisions for this rule are effective April 1, 2011.

B. Policy: The CY 2011 Final Rule for Home Health included requirements related to how and when therapy services are to be provided in the home health setting as well as documentation requirements for these visits. Policy details are provided in the above-mentioned chapter and summarized below.

II. BUSINESS REQUIREMENTS TABLE

Use "Shall" to denote a mandatory requirement

Number	Requirement	A / B MAC	D M E MAC	F I	C A R R I E R	R H H I	FISS	MCS	VMS	CWF	OTHER
							Shared-System Maintainers				
7374.1	Medicare contractors shall make providers aware of the clarifications provided in the updated manual sections attached to this instruction. A summary of these clarifications includes the following requirements: (1) assessment, measurement and documentation by occupational and physical therapists as well as speech-language pathologists (SLP) when providing therapy services in home health settings as specified in section 40.2.1and (2) qualified therapists rather than therapy assistants for occupational and physical therapy services must provide assessments for visits at specific intervals as specified in sections 40.2.1, 40.2.2, and 40.2.4.1. (This does not include speech-language pathology services only because SLP assistants are not recognized as providers for the home health benefit.)	X		X		X					

III. PROVIDER EDUCATION TABLE

Number	Requirement	Responsibility (place an "X" in each applicable column)									
		A/B MAC	DME MAC	FI	CARRIER	RHHI	FISS	MCS	VMS	CWF	OTHER
							Shared-System Maintainers				
7374.2	A provider education article related to this instruction will be available at http://www.cms.hhs.gov/MLNMattersArticles/ shortly after the CR is released. You will receive notification of the article release via the established "MLN Matters" listserv. Contractors shall post this article, or a direct link to this article (and the associated URL for the IOM), on their Web sites and include information about it in a listserv message within one week of the availability of the provider education article. In addition, the provider education article shall be included in the Contractors next regularly scheduled bulletin. Contractors are free to supplement MLN Matters articles with localized information (including the URL for the IOM) that would benefit their provider community in billing and administering the Medicare program correctly.	X		X		X					

IV. SUPPORTING INFORMATION

Section A: For any recommendations and supporting information associated with listed requirements, use the box below:
Use "Should" to denote a recommendation.

X-Ref Requirement Number	Recommendations or other supporting information:
N/A	

Section B: For all other recommendations and supporting information, use this space: N/A

V. CONTACTS

Pre-Implementation Contact(s): Kim Y. Evans, kim.evans@cms.hhs.gov or (410) 786-0009

Post-Implementation Contact(s): Contact your Contracting Officer's Technical Representative (COTR) or Contractor Manager, as applicable.

202   The How-to Guide to Home Health Therapy Documentation

VI. FUNDING

Section A: *For Fiscal Intermediaries (FIs), Regional Home Health Intermediaries (RHHIs),* **and/or** *Carriers***:**

No additional funding will be provided by CMS; contractor activities are to be carried out within their operating budgets.

Section B: *For Medicare Administrative Contractors (MACs)***:**

The Medicare Administrative Contractor is hereby advised that this constitutes technical direction as defined in your contract. CMS does not construe this as a change to the MAC Statement of Work. The contractor is not obligated to incur costs in excess of the amounts allotted in your contract unless and until specifically authorized by the contracting officer. If the contractor considers anything provided, as described above, to be outside the current scope of work, the contractor shall withhold performance on the part(s) in question and immediately notify the contracting officer, in writing or by e-mail, and request formal directions regarding continued performance requirements.

40.1.2.1 - Observation and Assessment of the Patient's Condition When Only the Specialized Skills of a Medical Professional Can Determine Patient's Status
(Rev.142, Issued: 04-15-11, Effective: 04-01-11, Implementation: 05-05-11)

Observation and assessment of the patient's condition by a nurse are reasonable and necessary skilled services whe*re there is a reasonable potential for* change in a patient's condition *that* requires skilled nursing personnel to identify and evaluate the patient's need for possible modification of treatment or initiation of additional medical procedures until the patient's treatment regimen is essentially stabilized. Where a patient was admitted to home health care for skilled observation because there was a reasonable potential of a complication or further acute episode, but did not develop a further acute episode or complication, the skilled observation services are still covered for *3* weeks or *so* long as there remains a reasonable potential for such a complication or further acute episode.

Information from the patient's medical history may support *whether there is a reasonable potential for* a future complication or acute episode and, therefore, may justify the need for continued skilled observation and assessment beyond *the* 3-week period. Moreover, such indications as abnormal/fluctuating vital signs, weight changes, edema, symptoms of drug toxicity, abnormal/fluctuating lab values, and respiratory changes on auscultation may justify skilled observation and assessment. Where these indications are such that *there is a reasonable potential* that skilled observation and assessment by a licensed nurse will result in changes to the treatment of the patient, then the services would be covered. There are cases where patients *whose condition may appear to be stable* continue to require skilled observation and assessment. (See examples below.) However, observation and assessment by a nurse is not reasonable and necessary to the treatment of the illness or injury where these indications are part of a longstanding pattern of the patient's condition *which itself does not require skilled services* and there is no attempt to change the treatment to resolve them.

EXAMPLE 1:

A patient with atherosclerotic heart disease with congestive heart failure requires observation by skilled nursing personnel for signs of decompensation or adverse effects resulting from prescribed medication. Skilled observation is needed to determine whether the drug regimen should be modified or whether other therapeutic measures should be considered until the patient's treatment regimen is essentially stabilized.

EXAMPLE 2:

A patient has undergone peripheral vascular disease treatment including a revascularization procedure (bypass). The incision area is showing signs of potential infection (e.g., heat, redness, swelling, drainage) and the patient has elevated body temperature. Skilled observation and monitoring of the vascular supply of the legs and the incision site is required until the signs of potential infection have abated and there is no longer a reasonable potential of infection.

EXAMPLE 3:

A patient was hospitalized following a heart attack, and following treatment but before mobilization, is discharged home. Because it is not known whether exertion will exacerbate the heart disease, skilled observation is reasonable and necessary as mobilization is initiated until the patient's treatment regimen is essentially stabilized.

EXAMPLE 4:

A frail 85-year old man was hospitalized for pneumonia. The infection was resolved, but the patient, who had previously maintained adequate nutrition, will not eat or eats poorly. The patient is discharged to the HHA for monitoring of fluid and nutrient intake and assessment of the need for tube feeding. Observation and monitoring by skilled nurses of the patient's oral intake, output and hydration status is required to determine what further treatment or other intervention is needed.

EXAMPLE 5:

A patient with glaucoma and a cardiac condition has a cataract extraction. Because of the interaction between the eye drops for the glaucoma and cataracts and the beta-blocker for the cardiac condition, the patient is at risk for serious cardiac arrhythmia. Skilled observation and monitoring of the drug actions is reasonable and necessary until the patient's condition is stabilized.

EXAMPLE 6:

A patient with hypertension suffered dizziness and weakness. The physician found that the blood pressure was too low and discontinued the hypertension medication. Skilled observation and monitoring of the patient's blood pressure and medication regimen is required until the blood pressure remains stable and in a safe range.

40.2.1 - General Principles Governing Reasonable and Necessary Physical Therapy, Speech-Language Pathology Services, and Occupational Therapy
(Rev. 142, Issued: 04-15-11, Effective: 04-01-11, Implementation: 05-05-11)

The service of a physical therapist, speech-language pathologist, or occupational therapist is a skilled therapy service if the inherent complexity of the service is such that it can be performed safely and/or effectively only by or under the general supervision of a skilled therapist. To be covered, the skilled services must also be reasonable and necessary to the treatment of the patient's illness or injury or to the restoration or maintenance of function affected by the patient's illness or injury. It is necessary to determine whether individual therapy services are skilled and whether, in view of the patient's overall condition, skilled management of the services provided is needed.

The development, implementation, management, and evaluation of a patient care plan based on the physician's orders constitute skilled therapy services when, because of the patient's condition, those activities require the skill*s of a qualified* therapist to *ensure the effectiveness of the treatment goals* and ensure medical safety. Where the skills of a therapist are needed to manage and periodically reevaluate the appropriateness of a maintenance program because of an identified danger to the patient, such services would be covered, even if the skills of a therapist were not needed to carry out the activities performed as part of the maintenance program.

While a patient's particular medical condition is a valid factor in deciding if skilled therapy services are needed, a patient's diagnosis or prognosis should never be the sole factor in deciding that a service is or is not skilled. The key issue is whether the skills of a therapist are needed to treat the illness or injury, or whether the services can be carried out by nonskilled personnel.

A service that is ordinarily considered nonskilled could be considered a skilled therapy service in cases in which there is clear documentation that, because of special medical complications, skilled rehabilitation personnel are required to perform the service. However, the importance of a particular service to a patient or the frequency with which it must be performed does not, by itself, make a nonskilled service into a skilled service.

The skilled therapy services must be reasonable and necessary to the treatment of the patient's illness or injury within the context of the patient's unique medical condition. To be considered reasonable and necessary for the treatment of the illness or injury:

a. The services must be consistent with the nature and severity of the illness or injury, the patient's particular medical needs, including the requirement that the amount, frequency, and duration of the services must be reasonable*; and*

b. The services must be considered, under accepted standards of medical practice, to be specific, safe, and effective treatment for the patient's condition, *meeting the standards noted below.*

1. *Assessment, Measurement and Documentation of Therapy Effectiveness*

To ensure therapy services are effective, at defined points during a course of treatment, for each therapy discipline for which services are provided, a qualified therapist (instead of an assistant) must perform the ordered therapy service. During this visit, the therapist must assess the patient using a method which allows for objective measurement of function and successive comparison of measurements. The therapist must document the measurement results in the clinical record. Specifically:

i. *Initial Therapy Assessment*

- *For each therapy discipline for which services are provided, a qualified therapist (instead of an assistant) must assess the patient's function using a method which objectively measures activities of daily living such as, but not limited to, eating, swallowing, bathing, dressing, toileting, walking, climbing stairs, using assistive devices, and mental and cognitive factors. The measurement results must be documented in the clinical record.*

- *Where more than one discipline of therapy is being provided, a qualified therapist from each of the disciplines must functionally assess the patient. The therapist must document the measurement results which correspond to the therapist's discipline and care plan goals in the clinical record.*

ii. *Reassessment at least every 30 days (performed in conjunction with an ordered therapy service)*

- *At least once every 30 days, for each therapy discipline for which services are provided, a qualified therapist (instead of an assistant) must provide the ordered therapy service, functionally reassess the patient, and compare the resultant measurement to prior assessment measurements. The therapist must document in the clinical record the measurement results along with the therapist's determination of the effectiveness of therapy, or lack thereof. The 30-day clock begins with the first therapy service (of that discipline) and the clock resets with each therapist's visit/assessment/measurement/ documentation (of that discipline).*

- *Where more than one discipline of therapy is being provided, at least once every 30 days, a qualified therapist from each of the disciplines must provide the ordered therapy service, functionally reassess the patient, and compare the resultant measurement to prior assessment measurements. The therapist must document in the clinical record the measurement results along with the therapist's determination of the effectiveness of therapy, or lack thereof. In multi-discipline therapy cases, the qualified therapist would reassess functional items (and measure and document) those which correspond to the therapist's discipline and care plan goals. In cases where more than one discipline of therapy is being provided, the 30-day clock begins with the first therapy service (of that discipline) and the clock resets with each therapist's visit/assessment/measurement/documentation (of that discipline).*

iii. *Reassessment prior to the 14th and 20th therapy visit*

- *If a patient's course of therapy treatment reaches 13 therapy visits, for each therapy discipline for which services are provided, a qualified therapist (instead of an assistant) must provide the ordered 13th therapy service, functionally reassess the patient, and compare the resultant measurement to prior measurements. The therapist must document in the clinical record the measurement results along with the therapist's determination of the effectiveness of therapy, or lack thereof.*

- *Similarly, if a patient's course of therapy treatment reaches 19 therapy visits, a qualified therapist (instead of an assistant) must provide the ordered 19th therapy service, functionally reassess, measure and document effectiveness of therapy, or lack thereof.*

- *When the patient resides in a rural area or when documented circumstances outside the control of the therapist prevent the qualified therapist's visit at exactly the 13th visit, the qualified therapist's visit can occur after the 10th therapy visit but no later than the 13th visit. Similarly, in rural areas or if documented exceptional circumstances exist, the qualified therapist's visit can occur after the 16th therapy visit but no later than the 19th therapy.*

- *Where more than one discipline of therapy is being provided, a qualified therapist from each of the disciplines must provide the ordered therapy service and functionally reassess, measure, and document the effectiveness of therapy or lack thereof close to but no later than the 13th and 19th therapy visit. The 13th and 19th therapy visit timepoints relate to the sum total of therapy visits from all therapy disciplines. In multi-discipline therapy cases, the qualified therapist would reassess functional items and measure those which correspond to the therapist's discipline and care plan goals.*

- *Therapy services provided after the 13th and 19th visit (sum total of therapy visits from all therapy disciplines), are not covered until:*

  The qualified therapist(s) completes the assessment/measurement/documentation requirements.

  The qualified therapist(s) determines if the goals of the plan of care have been achieved or if the plan of care may require updating. If needed, changes to therapy goals or an updated plan of care is sent to the physician for signature or discharge.

If the measurement results do not reveal progress toward therapy goals and/or do not indicate that therapy is effective, but therapy continues, the qualified therapist(s) must document why the physician and therapist have determined therapy should be continued.

c. Services involving activities for the general welfare of any patient, e.g., general exercises to promote overall fitness or flexibility and activities to provide diversion or general motivation do not constitute skilled therapy. Nonskilled individuals without the supervision of a therapist can perform those services.

d. *In order for therapy services to be covered, one of the following three conditions must be met:*

1. *The skills of a qualified therapist are needed to restore patient function:*

    - *To meet this coverage condition, therapy* services must be provided with the expectation, based on the assessment made by the physician of the patient's *restorative* potential that the condition of the patient will improve materially in a reasonable and generally predictable period of time. *Improvement is evidenced by objective successive measurements.*

    - *Therapy is not considered reasonable and necessary under this condition if the patient's expected restorative potential would be insignificant in relation to the extent and duration of therapy services required to reach such potential.*

    - *Therapy is not required to effect improvement or restoration of function where a patient suffers a transient or easily reversible loss of function (such as temporary weakness following surgery) which could reasonably be expected to improve spontaneously as the patient gradually resumes normal activities. Therapy in such cases is not considered reasonable and necessary to treat the patient's illness or injury, under this condition. However, if the criteria for maintenance therapy described in (3) below is met, therapy could be covered under that condition.*

2. *The patient's condition requires a qualified therapist to design or establish a maintenance program:*

    - *If the patient's clinical condition requires the specialized skill, knowledge and judgment of a qualified therapist to design or establish a maintenance program, related to the patient's illness or injury, in order to ensure the safety of the patient and the effectiveness of the program, such services are covered.*

    - *During the last visit(s) for restorative treatment, the qualified therapist may develop a maintenance program. The goals of a maintenance program would be, for example, to maintain functional status or to prevent decline in function.*

- *Periodic reevaluations of the beneficiary and adjustments to a maintenance program may be covered if such requires the specialized skills of a qualified therapist.*

- *Where a maintenance program is not established until after the rehabilitative therapy program has been completed, or where there was no rehabilitative therapy program, a qualified therapist's development of a maintenance program would be considered reasonable and necessary for the treatment of the patient's condition only when an identified danger to the patient exists.*

- *When designing or establishing a maintenance program, the qualified therapist must teach* the patient or the patient's family or caregiver's necessary techniques, exercises or precautions *as necessary* to treat the illness or injury. However, visits made by skilled therapists to a patient's home solely to train other HHA staff (e.g., home health aides) are not billable as visits since the HHA is responsible for ensuring that its staff is properly trained to perform any service it furnishes. The cost of a skilled therapist's visit for the purpose of training HHA staff is an administrative cost to the agency.

3. *The skills of a qualified therapist are needed to perform maintenance therapy:*

   Where the clinical condition of the patient is such that the complexity of the therapy services required to maintain function involve the use of complex and sophisticated therapy procedures to be delivered by the therapist himself/herself (and not an assistant) or the clinical condition of the patient is such that the complexity of the therapy services required to maintain function must be delivered by the therapist himself/herself (and not an assistant) in order to ensure the patient's safety and to provide an effective maintenance program, then those reasonable and necessary services should be covered.

e. The amount, frequency, and duration of the services must be reasonable.

40.2.2 - Application of the Principles to Physical Therapy Services
(Rev. 142, Issued: 04-15-11, Effective: 04-01-11, Implementation: 05-05-11)

The following discussion of skilled physical therapy services applies the principles in §40.2.1 to specific physical therapy services about which questions are most frequently raised.

A. Assessment

The skills of a physical therapist to assess and periodically reassess a patient's rehabilitation needs and potential or to develop and/or implement a physical therapy program are covered when they are reasonable and necessary because of the patient's condition. Skilled rehabilitation services concurrent with the management of a patient's care plan include objective tests and measurements such as, but not limited to, range of motion, strength, balance, coordination, endurance, or functional ability.

As described in section 40.2.1(b), at defined points during a course of therapy, the qualified physical therapist (instead of an assistant) must perform the ordered therapy service visit, assess the patient's function using a method which allows for objective measurement of function and comparison of successive measurements, and document the results of the assessments, corresponding measurements, and effectiveness of the therapy in the patient's clinical record. Refer to §40.2.1(b) for specific timing and documentation requirements associated with these requirements.

B. Therapeutic Exercises

Therapeutic exercises, which *require the skills of a* qualified physical therapist to ensure the safety of the beneficiary and the effectiveness of the treatment constitute skilled physical therapy, *when the criteria in §40.2.1(d) above are met.*

C. Gait Training

Gait evaluation and training furnished *to* a patient whose ability to walk has been impaired by neurological, muscular or skeletal abnormality require the skills of a qualified physical therapist and constitute skilled physical therapy and are considered reasonable and necessary if they can be expected to materially improve the patient's ability to walk. Gait evaluation and training which is furnished to a patient whose ability to walk has been impaired by a condition other than a neurological, muscular, or skeletal abnormality would nevertheless be covered where physical therapy is reasonable and necessary to restore *function. Refer to §40.2.1(d)(1) for the reasonable and necessary coverage criteria associated with restoring patient function.*

EXAMPLE 1:

A physician has ordered gait evaluation and training for a patient whose gait has been materially impaired by scar tissue resulting from burns. Physical therapy services to evaluate the beneficiary's gait, establish a gait training program, and provide the skilled services necessary to implement the program would be covered.

EXAMPLE 2:

A patient who has had a total hip replacement is ambulatory but demonstrates weakness and is unable to climb stairs safely. Physical therapy would be reasonable and necessary to teach the patient to climb and descend stairs safely.

Repetitive exercises to improve gait or to maintain strength and endurance and assistive walking are appropriately provided by nonskilled persons and ordinarily do not require the skills of a physical therapist. Where such services are performed by a physical therapist as part of the initial design and establishment of a safe and effective maintenance program, the services would, to the extent that they are reasonable and necessary *as defined in §40.2.1(d)(2),* be covered.

EXAMPLE 3:

A patient who has received gait training has reached their maximum restoration potential, and the physical therapist is teaching the patient and family how to safely perform the activities that are a part of the maintenance program. The visits by the physical therapist to demonstrate and teach the activities (which by themselves do not require the skills of a therapist) would be covered since they are needed to establish the program *(refer to §40.2.1(d)(2)).*

D. Range of Motion

Only a qualified physical therapist may perform range of motion tests and, therefore, such tests are skilled physical therapy.

Range of motion exercises constitute skilled physical therapy only if they are part of an active treatment for a specific disease state, illness, or injury that has resulted in a loss or restriction of mobility (as evidenced by physical therapy notes showing the degree of motion lost and the degree to be restored). Nonskilled individuals may provide range of motion exercises unrelated to the restoration of a specific loss of function often safely and effectively. Passive exercises to maintain range of motion in paralyzed extremities that can be carried out by nonskilled persons do not constitute skilled physical therapy.

However, *if the criteria in §40.2.1(d)(3) are met,* where there is clear documentation that, because of special medical complications (e.g., susceptible to pathological bone fractures), the skills of a therapist are needed to provide services which ordinarily do not need the skills of a therapist, and then the services would be covered.

E. Maintenance Therapy

Where repetitive services that are required to maintain function involve the use of complex and sophisticated procedures, the judgment and skill of a physical therapist might be required for the safe and effective rendition of such services. If the judgment and skill of a physical therapist *are* required to safely and effectively treat the illness or injury, the services would be covered as physical therapy services. *Refer to §40.2.1(d)(3).*

EXAMPLE 4:

Where there is an unhealed, unstable fracture that requires regular exercise to maintain function until the fracture heals, the skills of a physical therapist would be needed to ensure that the fractured extremity is maintained in proper position and alignment during maintenance range of motion exercises.

Establishment of a maintenance program is a skilled physical therapy service where the specialized knowledge and judgment of a qualified physical therapist is required for the program to be safely carried out and the treatment of the physician to be achieved.

EXAMPLE 5:

A Parkinson's patient or a patient with rheumatoid arthritis who has not been under a restorative physical therapy program may require the services of a physical therapist to determine what type of exercises are required to maintain the patient's present level of function. The initial evaluation of the patient's needs, the designing of a maintenance program appropriate to their capacity and tolerance and the treatment objectives of the physician, the instruction of the patient, family or caregivers to carry out the program safely and effectively and such reevaluations as may be required by the patient's condition, would constitute skilled physical therapy.

While a patient is under a restorative physical therapy program, the physical therapist should regularly reevaluate the patient's condition and adjust any exercise program the patient is expected to carry out alone or with the aid of supportive personnel to maintain the function being restored. Consequently, by the time it is determined that no further restoration is possible (i.e., by the end of the last restorative session) the physical therapist will already have designed the maintenance program required and instructed the patient or caregivers in carrying out the program.

F. Ultrasound, Shortwave, and Microwave Diathermy Treatments

These treatments must always be performed by or under the supervision of a qualified physical therapist and are skilled therapy.

G. Hot Packs, Infra-Red Treatments, Paraffin Baths and Whirlpool Baths

Heat treatments and baths of this type ordinarily do not require the skills of a qualified physical therapist. However, the skills, knowledge, and judgment of a qualified physical therapist might be required in the giving of such treatments or baths in a particular case, e.g., where the patient's condition is complicated by circulatory deficiency, areas of desensitization, open wounds, fractures, or other complications.

H. Wound Care Provided Within Scope of State Practice Acts

If wound care falls within the auspice of a physical therapist's State Practice Act, then the physical therapist may provide the specific type of wound care services defined in the

State Practice Act. *However, such visits in this specific situation would be a covered therapy service only when the skills of a therapist are required to perform the service.*

40.2.3 - Application of the General Principles to Speech-Language Pathology Services
(Rev. 142, Issued: 04-15-11, Effective: 04-01-11, Implementation: 05-05-11)

The following discussion of skilled speech-language pathology services applies the principles to specific speech-language pathology services about which questions are most frequently raised.

As described in §40.2.1(b), at defined points during a course of therapy, the qualified speech-language pathologist must perform the ordered therapy service visit, assess the patient's function using a method which allows for objective measurement of function and comparison of successive measurements, and document the results of the assessments, corresponding measurements, and effectiveness of therapy in the patient's clinical record. Refer to §40.2.1(b) for specific timing and documentation requirements associated with these requirements.

1. The skills of a speech-language pathologist are required for the assessment of a patient's rehabilitation needs (including the causal factors and the severity of the speech and language disorders), and rehabilitation potential. Reevaluation would be considered reasonable and necessary only if the patient exhibited:

    - A change in functional speech or motivation;

    - Clearing of confusion; or

    - The remission of some other medical condition that previously contraindicated speech-language pathology services.

    Where a patient is undergoing restorative speech-language pathology services, routine reevaluations are considered to be a part of the therapy and cannot be billed as a separate visit.

2. The services of a speech-language pathologist would be covered if they are needed as a result of an illness or injury and are directed towards specific speech/voice production.

3. Speech-language pathology would be covered where the service can only be provided by a speech-language pathologist and where it is reasonably expected that the service will materially improve the patient's ability to independently carry out any one or combination of communicative activities of daily living in a manner that is measurably at a higher level of attainment than that prior to the initiation of the services.

4. The services of a speech-language pathologist to establish a hierarchy of speech-voice-language communication tasks and cueing that directs a patient toward speech-language communication goals in the plan of care would be covered speech-language pathology.

5. The services of a speech-language pathologist to train the patient, family, or other caregivers to augment the speech-language communication, treatment, or to establish an effective maintenance program would be covered speech-language pathology services.

6. The services of a speech-language pathologist to assist patients with aphasia in rehabilitation of speech and language skills are covered when needed by a patient.

7. The services of a speech-language pathologist to assist patients with voice disorders to develop proper control of the vocal and respiratory systems for correct voice production are covered when needed by a patient.

40.2.4.1 - Assessment
(Rev. 142, Issued: 04-15-11, Effective: 04-01-11, Implementation: 05-05-11)

The skills of an occupational therapist to assess and reassess a patient's rehabilitation needs and potential or to develop and/or implement an occupational therapy program are covered when they are reasonable and necessary because of the patient's condition.

As described in §40.2.1(b), at defined points during a course of therapy, the qualified occupational therapist (instead of an assistant) must perform the ordered therapy service visit, assess the patient's function using a method which allows for objective measurement of function and comparison of successive measurements, and document the results of the assessments, corresponding measurements, and effectiveness of therapy in the patient's clinical record. Refer to §40.2.1(b) for specific timing and documentation requirements associated with these requirements.